SEX, SIN,
AND
SALVATION

SEX, SIN,
AND
SALVATION

RICHARD HANSON, M.ED., L.P.

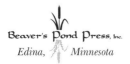

Beaver's Pond Press, Inc.
Edina, Minnesota

ISBN 1-931646-55-4

Library of Congress Catalog Number: 2002107410

Printed in the United States of America

First Printing: November 2002

06 05 04 03 02   6 5 4 3 2 1

Beaver's Pond Press, Inc.   5125 Danen's Drive
Edina, MN 55439-1465
(952) 829-8818
www.beaverspondpress.com

to order, visit *midwestbookhouse.com* or call 1-877-430-0044. Quantity discounts available.

*This book is dedicated
to my children, M. & L.,
and my wife, P.*

ACKNOWLEDGEMENTS

I would like to thank the following individuals and groups for their support in the preparation of this book: Cheryl Ostlund, Rabbi Barry Woolf, Rachel Lasky, Mori Studio, Richard Swenson, and Editor Douglas Benson.

TABLE OF CONTENTS

.

PREFACE

When I began to plan this book I had been struggling with the issues of sexuality and guilt for many years. Setting these issues down on paper has helped me grow as a person. My views have expanded and have come to encompass a much larger view of human sexuality. I have found a much greater acceptance of my sexuality and discovered a way to lift the burden of guilt from my own life. I believe this process is worth sharing with others. I realize there is more to say than what I say in these pages. This is perhaps just the beginning of the dialogue. It is my hope that clergy will use this book as a springboard for discussion of sexuality in the churches and synagogues. Sexuality is best discussed in all of its aspects: physical, emotional and spiritual. Let us begin!

R.H.

CHAPTER I

SEXUAL REPRESSION AND GUILT

THE SEXUALITY OF JESUS

Jesus, according to Christian doctrine, was both divine and human, fully God and fully man—God in human form. As a human, he was subject to the full range of human experience and temptations, no doubt including sexual temptation.

Being human, Jesus probably entered his teenage years with the increasing awareness of human—and his own—sexuality common to adolescence.

As an adult, Jesus may have been attracted to women, like any healthy male. The sexuality of Jesus is not discussed in the Bible. I think this is because the writers were uncomfortable with the topic, and this discomfort has persisted to our present day. This has caused humans immense difficulties. I am writing this book to bring some balance to our view of sexuality.

As Jesus lived his life, He doubtless thought about what was most important. He longed for a home and most certainly had thoughts of a wife and the joys of intimacy. In Matthew 8:20 we read: *"...and Jesus said to him, 'Foxes have holes and birds of the air have nests, but the Son of man has nowhere to lay his head.'"* This clearly reveals the humanity of the Lord as one who longed for the care that a person can experience only in a family. Organized religion has emphasized the divinity of Jesus and denied His humanness. I believe this is because religious leaders realize that to deal with His humanity they must come to terms with Him as a sexual being and they don't know how to do it. It is not as scary as it seems. All we have to do is face the fact that Christ was human and a sexual being and that is all right. When we do this, we can come to a realization that it is acceptable for us to be sexual.

The traditional teaching in religion portrays Jesus as a person who denied His sexuality and remained a virgin throughout His life. This is not stated in the Bible; it is an assumption on the part of religious leaders. When one examines this teaching, it does make sense. When you look at the life of Christ, it is crystal clear that He lived it with total integrity. It seems reasonable then to expect that if He had a sexual relationship it would be in the context of a loving marriage. He would not have gone around having casual sex. If he was married, he could not have been saying that He had "nowhere to lay his head."

Jesus could have remained a virgin and still could have been tempted to have sexual relationships; perhaps with Mary Magdalene. He was subjected to all of the temptations known to humans, after all. The very idea of Jesus having thoughts about sex will be a source of consternation to many clergy. They often are ill at ease with their own sexuality and, as a result, have considerable difficulty talking about sexuality with the members of their congregations.

HOW DID WE GET INTO THIS MESS?

None of us was born with guilty feelings about our sexual nature. We had to be taught to be uncomfortable with it. Unfortunately, many of us were taught in our house of worship to think of sex as shameful. This is the sad legacy of our encounter with the most basic part of our nature in a theological context. It is time to change! This change must begin with the members of the clergy. Many need to learn to become free of the guilt binding them to the past.

The prevalent mindset among many religious leaders sees sex itself as evil. One source for this idea is probably Psalm 51:5: *"I was brought forth in iniquity and in sin did my mother conceive me."* Obviously, "my mother conceived me," as a result of the act of sexual intercourse. In this context it is easy to conclude that sexual intercourse itself is sinful. I believe this is actually what has happened among many religious leaders. They have a tremendous dilemma here. We are by nature sexual beings, and if our sexuality is inherently evil then we are inherently evil. If this is not the case, then we must see our sexuality as good, as positive. I believe that our sexuality is positive. After all, this is the way God created us.

Psalm 51:5 indicates the presence of sin in the lives of my mother and father; therefore, I was conceived by two people who were less than perfect. But, the act of sexual intercourse involving a husband and wife is no more inherently sinful than any other act humans engage in during their lives.

PLEASURE AND CHRISTIANITY

Christian churches tend to handle the concept of pleasure, especially sexual pleasure, rather poorly. This may be a result of the way Jesus and His contemporaries are portrayed in the Bible: Jesus comes across as someone who was called to a life of suffering and never had any fun. I refuse to accept this picture as accurate. I believe that Christ experienced joy and pleasure in His life. He must have played games, told jokes, laughed and been lighthearted. However, He is rarely presented this way in scripture. I think this says a lot about the writers of the New Testament. They must have been a depressed and depressing group. A clear exception is the writer of the Song of Solomon, of which I will speak later.

Psychotherapy

A sense of humor is one of the most important characteristics humans possess. People with a good sense of humor cope much better with life that those who have a poor sense of humor. In fact, I have worked with people who have almost no sense of humor at all and they seem to be like zombies, like the living dead. For this reason, I am convinced that Jesus had a sense of humor because He was a healthy human being.

Pleasure as Positive

When the Christian church can accept pleasure as positive it can come to terms with sexual behavior. It can then acknowledge that pleasure is an important and desirable part of sexuality. This will become easier when religious leaders come to see sexual pleasure as a gift from God. One step toward this end is to see Christ as human and capable of sensual gratification.

Sexual union not only satisfies our physical senses but, in the context of love, also meets our spiritual needs. There is something mysterious, beyond human telling, when two become one flesh. It is not necessary to understand it, all one has to do is accept it. This is why the love between a husband and wife is deeper than any other love between humans. Within the bonds of marriage we can experience the love of God.

Orgasm

Human beings were created to have orgasms. It is the most intense ecstasy that we as human beings experience. I believe people should have all the sexual climaxes that they can. Clergy, for the most part, are uncomfortable with their own sexuality and have a great deal of fear of even discussing it. In the survey I conducted, most respondents had no idea where their church stands on questions about sexual behavior. They said that there is no discussion of sexual issues in their place of worship. People continue to seek sexual pleasure, but they do it in a moral vacuum. They don't know if they should feel guilty about their activity or not. They seem to have lingering guilt and shame about it. One of my goals in writing this book is to lift the burden of sex-related guilt from people's lives so they can enjoy greater freedom and happiness.

A DEFINITION OF LOVE

> *"Love is patient and kind, never jealous or envious, never boastful or proud, never haughty or selfish, or rude. Love does not demand its own way."*
>
> **I Corinthians 13:4-5**

This Biblical quote is a good starting place when constructing a definition of love. It is in contradiction to the images of love that are reflected in our culture through popular music, television, and movies. Jealousy is thought to be a sign of love. When a person sees his or her loved one with another woman or man, it is common for this person to be jealous. One may even be jealous of the time his or her loved one spends working because this represents time away from their togetherness. But, is this really love? If it is, is it healthy love? I don't think so.

Extreme jealousy is a sign that one person is very dependent upon the other. Dependence can become pathological. Indeed, some people become addicted to another person much as some become addicted to chemicals. This is not love, and it is not healthy.

In a truly loving relationship each individual has a lot of freedom. The two people involved enjoy being together and doing things together, but they realize that they have separate interests and other friends with whom they also want to do things. When two lovers have experiences with others it enriches their relationship by providing new ideas for them to share. Many relationships flounder because of boredom when there is no input from the outside.

"Love does not demand its own way." The issue that springs readily to mind is one of sexual desire. When a boy or young man is seriously attracted to a girl or young woman, sexual desire arises. That desire becomes easily confused with love. If he loves her, he will not demand his own way. When he demands that she "prove" her love for him, this is manipulation and exploitation of the female by the male. Nothing could be further from love. In addition to manipulating her and devaluing sex, he is also placing her in the position of risking pregnancy. This, if she is a teenager, could be a very traumatic experience for her and result in long-term suffering. This is not love!

I am convinced that many people do not know what love *is*. I don't claim to have the final answer, but I have some ideas about the subject that I would like to share. I believe that if you love someone, you want that person to be happy. You would like to see that person grow and develop to his or her fullest potential. If you love someone, you will be willing to sacrifice something yourself so that your loved one can achieve and grow.

A clear example of love is when parents adjust their lives in order to save enough money to send their children to college. It is common for parents to make sacrifices for their children because they love them. In fact, many people will go to considerable trouble to make their children happy. However, often they will not sacrifice much of anything for their spouse. I believe this is particularly true of men. Women seem to do more than half of the compromising in marriage.

Why is this? I believe that, in part, it has to do with an erroneous definition of masculinity. If a man works two jobs to provide money for his daughter's or son's education, he is seen as a good provider, in other words, as masculine. However, if he declines an invitation to play golf with the other men from the office because he has to go home and stay with his children so that his wife can go to her tennis match, he will probably be seen as henpecked, or lacking in masculinity. In reality, if he really loves his wife, he is willing to work out a schedule with her that accommodates both of their interests. He is just as manly when he is providing child-care as he is when playing golf with other men. Masculinity does not depend upon activity. Remember, also, all men have a feminine side to them, whether they acknowledge it or not. This in no way decreases their manliness. Instead it may very well enhance it.

> *"Love is never glad about injustice, but rejoices whenever truth wins out. If you love someone you will be loyal to him or her no matter what the cost. You will always believe in him or her, always expect the best of him or her, and always stand your ground in defending him or her"*
>
> **I Corinthians 13:6-7**

What a radical idea! To love someone is to stick with that person, come what may. In our time, when divorce rampant, it is apparent that this is not what people mean when they say, "I love you." We have "fair-weather lovers." As long as things are fairly comfortable, they will hang in there, but let things get a little rough, and they want out. This is not love and should not be considered as such.

I am not saying that people should remain married no matter what. There are relationships that have deteriorated to the point of no return, and divorce is the only logical alternative. What I am saying is that too many people have very unrealistic ideas about love and marriage. They want instant and perpetual happiness with little or no effort. Love and marriage are hard work! I strongly believe that this is what we need to teach our children. Open their eyes wide, before they marry. Then they may have a better chance at more long-lasting happiness.

LOVE AND LUST

Heterosexual men and women are, by design, sexually attracted to each other. In marriage, sexual attraction, sexual arousal, intercourse, and orgasm are healthy and normal. There is nothing wrong with this behavior in this context.

Many "religious" people have not fully accepted this and are still uncomfortable with sexuality, even in marriages.

There are many marriages in which one or both partners have lost interest in sex and in which there is no passion. Often a great load of guilt has finally overwhelmed their libido and some have become asexual. I think this is because many people confuse love and lust. Since lust is one of the seven deadly sins, it then becomes impossible to conceive of Jesus experiencing sexual attraction to females because He was righteous and without sin. Since Jesus was without blemish, He could not have been attracted to women, because lust is sinful. But love isn't the same as lust! This is another distortion of some theologies. Normal attraction between men and women is healthy and part of God's plan.

Lust is a different story. It is an overwhelming desire to possess. If its uncontrolled, the desire can become the master, not the person. The desire is manifested as an intense longing for sexual union with a particular person or persons. It is wanting to have sex with another person solely for the pursuit of pleasure and physical release. Lust leads to the objectification of one's partners and to a denial of their humanness.

In lust we see only the physical body of the other person and we are blind to his or her spiritual and emotional life. We treat the person as an object. Men, in particular, have viewed women as sex objects frequently. This behavior has been encouraged by the media in our society, particularly certain magazines that feature photographs of nude women. When a man looks at one of these photos, the woman becomes a sex object to him. He has no way to interact with her as a person, to know her as a human. He can only stare at her naked flesh and have sexual fantasies about her. Perhaps the worst part of lust is not the desire for sexual gratification, but rather that it reduces a precious human being to a mere object, a toy.

THE CATHOLIC CHURCH

I believe that the Roman Catholic Church has fomented a great deal of the guilt regarding sexuality. Consider their teachings and you will understand why I take this position. Catholics, like most Christian denominations, teach that Jesus was without sin and sexually abstinent. This is their model for males. The Catholic role model for females is the Virgin Mary. Their teaching has been that Mary was not only a virgin at the time of the birth of Jesus, but that she remained a virgin all of her life. Priests, the messengers of God within the Catholic Church, are expected to be sexually abstinent or asexual.

I think the idea of chastity for priests is a bad idea and runs contrary to human nature. It asks priests to deny an important aspect of their humanness, their sexuality. In fact, chastity has not been practiced by all those whom Catholics claim as their own. Peter, the ostensible founder of the papacy, was married and did not practice chastity.

I spoke with a priest about this, a man I will call Father Gabriel. He did acknowledge that Peter was married, but he didn't want to talk about it at any length. According to Father

Gabriel, the priesthood did not exist in the first century A.D. The early church followed the Jewish tradition. The idea of priestly celibacy is based largely on the writings of the Apostle Paul in I Corinthians. In this book we find Paul advising people who are single not to marry. This seems to be because he was expecting the second coming of Christ at any moment. Also, Paul was not urging only clergy to remain celibate, but all single people. This is inconsistent with Catholic doctrine where only the clergy must be celibate. As far as Father Gabriel knows there was no specific date on which celibacy became church doctrine. In his view the Council of Trent did affirm it as an official church teaching. There are former Episcopalian priests who are married and have returned to the Catholic Church and are working as Catholic priests. This is causing tension and concern within the church.

Father Gabriel and I did discuss the issue or ordination of women as priests. In his view if this were to occur it would cause major disruption within the Catholic Church. Many people would never accept it. They might leave the church. There is a particular concern about people in Latin cultures accepting women as priests. There is considerable fear that if women became priests, many Latin men would simply refuse to attend church anymore. Thus, the reasons for excluding women from the priesthood seem to be largely political.

The issue of Catholics keeping sexuality at arm's length remains, however. Mary and Jesus, as the female and male model, respectively, are portrayed as asexual. Priests are required to be, at least in theory, asexual. The idea that is conveyed through such practices is that those who acknowledge and enjoy their sexuality are somehow less revered in the Catholic Church and in the Kingdom of God than are those who are asexual.

Those who administer the sacraments, particularly communion, are the closest to God, and they cannot distribute the body and blood of Christ and be sexual. This restriction conveys and reinforces the notion that to be sexual is to be sinful.

I think they have gotten it completely wrong. Sexual activity is for the purpose of enhancing the relationship between partners through pleasure and ecstatic release. Conception is a bonus, if and when the partners want to avail themselves to this aspect of their sexual life. An increasing number of Catholics find some of the teachings of the their Church are not realistic and relevant to contemporary life; many of them are following practices not approved by the church.

This lessens the influence of the church in the everyday lives of many of its members. It also results in these people wandering in a perpetual desert of guilt, doubt and unhappiness.

I interviewed a Catholic Priest and asked him if teenagers in his church came to him with questions about whether they should become involved sexually with a boyfriend/girlfriend. His answer was no, they do not. I asked him why he thought this was the case. He said, "We have lost our prophetic vision."

I would take it one step beyond what he said and say that the Catholic Church has clung to a rigid, guilt-ridden outmoded view of sexual behavior.

Some people say that the prohibition against ordaining women as priests in the Catholic Church is because women menstruate. In the Old Testament, when a woman was having her period, she was seen as unclean. Being unclean, she would be unable to conduct the sacrament of communion. She could not distribute the body and blood of Christ in her unclean state. This is another larger layer of irrational and unsound guilt laid upon women by the Catholic Church.

Menstruation is a natural body function. Women were created by God to menstruate. It is out of the Old Testament that the idea has come that the makes them unclean, not out of the New Testament. Surely we know now that having her period does not make a woman unclean, so there is no reason that women can't be ordained in our time.

Catholic leaders take the position that because all of the apostles were male, they cannot ordain women. Yet Jesus never expressly prohibited the ordination of women. He never said that women cannot be ordained. Women's roles have changed since the time Jesus lived on earth. In His time, women were primarily homemakers, caring for children and tending to domestic activities. Men provided the primary support of the family. All this has changed. Today, women have taken their place in the world of work and have shown that they are as equally capable as men. Many Protestant denominations, including the Lutheran Church, did not ordain women throughout most of their history. Recently, however, noting the changing roles of women, they changed their policy. Female clergy in Protestant church bodies have not caused a lot of problems; in fact, their presence has improved the ministry. It is time for the Catholic Church to face the fact that times have changed.

I have written about the Catholic Church because of its pervasive influence. It has the most members of any Christian denomination in the United States, and it has a major impact in society. Its influence extends beyond its doors, and it has been responsible for sexual repression in our country even among non-Catholics.

PROTESTANT CHURCHES

Protestants don't fare much better, however. Teenagers in Protestant churches are not seeking the advice of their clergy as to whether or not they should begin to have sexual relations. The Protestant churches are not addressing the issue well—in fact, they are, for the most part, avoiding it. This is because of the overwhelming sense of shame that they feel about sexuality.

Most Protestant clergy are married, since they have no vow of chastity. One would expect that, being married they are sexually active, although this is not always the case because there are numerous marriages in which there is no physical intimacy. Guilt has invaded the bedroom to such an extent that some people, even in a loving marriage, cannot function sexually.

My goal is to free people from the chains of guilt and to let them be free as God intended.

ORAL-GENITAL SEX

In addressing the issue of sexual repression, the one thing that seems to cause the most anxiety among clergy is oral-genital sex. This is because the sex organs themselves are seen as dirty, nasty, unmentionable. If this is the case, how can one even think of putting one's mouth on your partner's organ? A school principal I know told me that a fifth grade boy said to a fifth-grade girl on the school bus, "Suck my nasty." In this simple phrase he captured the view of a great many "religious" people. If his penis is nasty, what would the girl be if she sucked it? Nasty, of course.

The word fellatio is interesting. It is defined as "to suck." and "Oral stimulation of the penis." It is not a word that has become popular. In the throes of passion, a woman seldom says to her partner, "How about a little fellatio?" One reason women don't say this is because many men wouldn't know what they were talking about! The common expression is to "go down on you." Cunnilingus is literally, "the act of licking" and secondarily, "oral stimulation of the vulva or clitoris." A man does not say to his lover, "how about some cunnilingus?" The common expression for a man to use is, "I'm going to lick you out." "Cunt," a slang term for the vagina, seems to have come from the word cunnilingus.

Many people are very uncomfortable with oral-genital sex. From my questionnaire and my own experience, it seems as if this is more common among older people. I received a questionnaire from a couple who where in their mid 70's. He was a college graduate and she had two years of college so they were highly educated. Their comments on oral-genital sex are, "We disapprove, no interest. It is unnatural and dangerous. I believe it is unnatural, unnecessary, unsanitary and spreads disease. Creates an atmosphere of immorality in a relationship."

Oral-genital sex is not for everyone. If people are uncomfortable with it, they should not practice it. However, it is important to separate the fact from fiction on this issue. The first thing I want to address is whether or not it is unnatural. This is probably the question that causes the most anxiety because most people equate doing something unnatural with being a pervert. People can do something kinky, but they don't want to practice what they might think is a perversion. Whether or not oral-genital sex is unnatural depends upon what a person thinks the primary purpose of sexual activity is. If you believe, as I do, that the main goal in having sex is pleasure, then it is not unnatural. Oral contact with the sex organ increases pleasure. Thus, it is natural extension of human behavior.

There is a common misconception that this type of love-making spreads disease. It can, if one or both partners have a sexually transmitted disease. But for healthy couples, it will not spread disease. It is expected that couples will bathe or shower before having sexual contact and thus will be clean and fresh. In regard to spreading disease, AIDS is more likely to be contracted through sexual intercourse than through oral-genital sex. One caution—herpes simplex, which, causes what are commonly called "cold sores" in the mouth, can be spread to the sex organ of one's partner during oral-genital lovemaking.

Another point raised by the elderly couple was that this type of sex creates an atmosphere of immortality in a relationship. But if behavior between two *consenting* adults brings them greater pleasure, strengthens the bond between them, and results in their experiencing greater happiness, how can it be immoral? To call it immoral is to restrict sexual behavior to a certain prescribed routine and is the enemy of freedom. Indeed, it is my experience as a sex therapist that most men and women want to have oral-genital sex. If their partner is unwilling to engage in this type of lovemaking, they will sometimes seek it out with prostitutes or other lovers. This is certainly immoral. I am not condoning extramarital sex so that people can have oral-genital sex; I am just stating what can happen in relationships.

This is one issue that should be clearly agreed upon when a couple gets married; i.e., are they or are they not going to have oral-genital sex? Many people believe they can change their partner after they are married, that the partner will come around. The person believes that even if a partner says that she/he doesn't want to have oral-genital sex, once we are married, he/she will be able to convince the partner to not only do it, but also to enjoy it. This is manipulation. Attempting to get one's partner to do what he or she doesn't want to do is an attempt to control the other person, which sets up an unequal relationship. Intimacy requires an equal relationship.

CHAPTER II

PERMISSION TO BE SEXUAL

God created us as sexual beings. We are free to be sexual with each other. In Genesis 1:27 it says, "So God created man in his own image, in the image of God he created him, male and female he created them." God is the highest authority, and He endorses our sexuality. In view of this, it may seem strange for people to feel as though they need permission to be sexual, but many do. Great numbers of people are uncomfortable with their bodies and have great difficulty communicating their sexual desires to their partners. This is because there is so much guilt intertwined with our view of sexuality.

Organized religion has been responsible for much of the guilt and shame that have been heaped on people regarding their sexual nature. As a result, religious bodies have lost credibility with many people and have also lost members. This is sad, because many people do not have a spiritual life once they leave a worshipping community. It is very important to have a spiritual life, but a spiritual life must embrace a full and fruitful sexual life. In fact, the act of intercourse between two people very much in love with one another is not only a physical experience, but a spiritual one also. This is what religious leaders have too often failed to understand. They have compartmentalized human beings, separating the life of the flesh. It is time to recognize the true nature of human existence, which is a unity, a whole.

Sexuality and Self-Esteem

Sexuality is a gift from God. Don't ever forget it! We were created to derive great pleasure from sexual union with another human being. This is part of the Divine Plan. Accept it, live it, enjoy it to the utmost, and respect it. Hold your head up; be comfortable with your sexuality, realizing that it is at your very core. See it as a gift for achieving intimacy, not as a way to exploit others. When you exploit others, you alienate yourself from God, others humans, and yourself. When you act in this way, you do not really respect yourself, and you destroy your self-esteem rather than building it. But when you have a reverence for life and treat your sexual nature and that of others' with respect, your self-esteem grows and peace comes to you.

What About Your Body?

In giving yourself permission to be sexual you will find it necessary to come to terms with your body. If you are uncomfortable with your body, you will be inhibited in your sexual expression and you will never experience the total ecstasy that is possible. If you don't like the way you look in the nude, your lover will sense this and the impact upon your relationship will be negative. To be at ease with your physical appearance, look at yourself, and see your body as it is. I recommend standing in front of a full-length mirror in the nude. When you do, rate yourself as follows:

1. Face and hair

   Excellent   Good   Fair

2. Breasts (female), Chest (male)

   Excellent   Good   Fair

3. Abdomen

   Excellent   Good   Fair

4. Pubic hair

   Excellent   Good   Fair

5. Vagina (female), Penis (male)

   Excellent   Good   Fair

6. Thighs

   Excellent   Good   Fair

7. Calves

   Excellent   Good   Fair

8. Feet and hands

   Excellent   Good   Fair

At this point turn around and look over your shoulder.

9. Back

   Excellent   Good   Fair

10. Buttocks (Derriere)

   Excellent   Good   Fair

I intentionally did not provide any guidelines as to what is excellent, good, or fair in regard to your appearance. I want you to trust your own judgment about your appearance. This exercise is designed to increase your comfort with your body, to enhance your self-esteem. It doesn't matter what others think; it matters only what *you* think. As you examine yourself, if there is something you don't like and you can change it, do it *now*. If you don't like your hairstyle, change it to a style that you do like. Whatever changes you make will increase your self-esteem and enhance your sexuality. Remember, not everyone wants the same thing in a sex partner's body, and there is someone in the world who will take you just as you are.

Take an honest look at your body. If you are very self-conscious when you first stand in front of the mirror, you may need to do it every day, increasing the time each day. If you do this over a few weeks, you will become more comfortable with your body. It's okay to take time to let this happen, there is no deadline. When you become at ease viewing your naked flesh, think about whether or not your assets outweigh your liabilities. If they do, celebrate this fact in some way that's meaningful to you. If you are overweight, give serious thought to what you want to do about it. Some people are attracted to large people—in fact, some men are attracted to "queen-sized" women, no matter what the media says. You may decide to seek romance at your current weight and, if you are totally comfortable with this decision, then go for it! On the other hand, you may decide you want to lose or gain weight. If you come to this position, there is on very important thing to keep in mind: be honest with yourself.

Don't Lie to Yourself

People who say they want to lose weight but do not do so are not telling the whole truth, not even to themselves. What they are saying is, if it was easy to lose weight, they would do it. But if it is difficult, they can't do it. If this is the case with you, admit it! Don't lie to yourself. If you are unwilling to learn and exercise the discipline required to achieve permanent weight loss, be honest with yourself and say so. I promise you will feel better when you do it. The discipline necessary for permanent weight loss must be learned. If you already knew how to exercise this discipline, you already would have achieved the weight reduction you desire. Since your weight is not what you want it to be, you clearly do not fully comprehend what's needed to change it. Oh, sure, you know something about discipline and self-control, but your program is incomplete. What is effective will be for you to completely change the way you think about food. I am not going to provide a program for you in this book. There is a wealth of information available to you from many sources. You can begin looking in your public library. So, turn off the TV, put aside your high-calorie, high-fat snacks, go out and get into your car and drive to the library. Do it now! If you think up an excuse not to take action, you will be more at peace with yourself if you admit that your desire for change is not great enough for you to take the action necessary. Just don't lie to yourself, because lying will lower your self-esteem.

STAGE II—INTIMACY WITH ONESELF

By this time you have viewed your body in the full-length mirror and become comfortable with seeing yourself naked. The next step is for you to touch your body, to become familiar with your own flesh. This may seem inappropriate to you, and you may have difficulty doing it. This is because of guilt and alienation you have experienced, and the origin of these feelings is probably in your religious training.

The way to overcome this guilt is through action. Touching "non-sexual" parts of your body is a good way to begin. Stroke your cheeks, your neck, your ears. When you do this you will discover what you enjoy. Then when you make love, telling your partner what you like will result in a much more fulfilling experience and will eliminate the guesswork and trial-by-error approach to lovemaking that can decrease desire.

Many people find it very erotic to have their partner kiss, suck on, blow into, or put their tongue in their ear. Obviously, you can't do this to yourself, but if, when stroking your ear with your fingers, you discover it is a sensuous experience, chances are you will enjoy oral stimulation of your ears by your partner. If this is the case, be sure to tell your partner to do this when you make love. Now touch your arms and stroke them lightly with your fingers. Do this to the back of your neck. Do you like it? Some people find it very sensuous to have their back stroked lightly by their partner.

Lie on the floor, take a full deep breath, hold you breath for a second, then exhale. Continue to breathe in this way. As you breathe slowly and deeply, be aware of your body and the sensations you experience. It is best if you do this in the nude. Be aware of how your body feels against the carpet you are lying on. Get in touch with the rhythm of your breathing, of your life! (It is an unfortunate fact that we too often lose touch with ourselves in our culture.

At this point, you are ready to move on. If you are a woman, stand in front of the mirror and look at your breasts. Be aware of your response to this experience. Touch them and be aware of how they feel. Think about how they fell to your partner. Ask him about his response to this part of your anatomy. (This is also a good opportunity for you to examine you breasts for any lumps or other abnormalities that might be a sign of cancer.)

Now, using a hand mirror, examine your vagina or penis. Look closely at the most intimate part of your physical/sexual being, your primary sex organ. Think about whether or not you think it is attractive. If your pubic hair is too long, you can always trim it a bit. Touch your vagina or penis. Become aware of what gives you the most pleasure in this regard. At the right moment, convey this information to your lover.

Cʀᴇᴀᴛɪɴɢ ᴀɴᴅ Aᴜʀᴀ ᴏꜰ Sᴇxᴜᴀʟɪᴛʏ

Plan to enhance and maximize your sexual experience. A good place to start is with what you are going to wear. The great majority of men are more attracted to and more aroused by a woman in sexy lingerie than by one who is sim- ply naked. Go shopping together so you both have input into what is purchased. See-through garments are generally the most exciting. A woman's breasts are much more tantalizing if they are partially covered, but still visible through the mate- rial. This experience drives some men wild! Perfume is also very important. Find out what scent your lover likes the best. Wear it in strategic places; besides putting it on your ears and wrists, try some between your breasts and your inner thighs.

Men, make sure you have had a shower and smell good! Tight-fitting jockey shorts bulging with one's manhood is a turn-on to many women. Many women find cologne may be as important to you as perfume is to your partner. Find out what scent she likes. Apply it not just to your face, but also to your chest and inner thighs.

Music will contribute significantly to an atmosphere of sensuality. Discuss your music selections between the two of you. For some people, a certain singer singing love songs will be a perfect background to their lovemaking. For others, instrumental pieces will be their choice. Experiment with different music until you find what you like best.

Generally, it is more desirable to have music playing softly in the background than to have it blasting at full volume. The choice is up to you, of course. Soft music enhances an atmosphere of intimacy between the two of you. A feeling of peace and mutual giving between the two of you will bring the greatest joy and highest points of ecstasy.

Lighting is very important. It has a significant impact upon the mood you create. I suggest undressing each other in the bright light. Looking at your partner's body is a pleasure available to you and one you should not pass up. You may begin to caress each other in the bright light. After a time, you may find it more sensual to dim the lights. Some couples prefer to be in darkness when they make love. If you are more comfortable in the dark, it's fine. Soft light allows you to still see your partner's body and also adds to the sense of mystery which surrounds our sexuality. Reduced lighting may increase your sense of romance and enhance your experience. You also can experiment with different colored lights. Just as vanilla is only one of the many flavors of ice cream available to us, so white is only one of the colors of light available. You can have red, purple, green, yellow, etc. You may even want to use a different color each season of the year or for each week of the month. The important thing is to try different approaches to lovemaking, to bring variety to your experience.

Place is important in your love life, too. Most couples make love in their bed. This is fine, but if it is the only place you ever have sex, your experience will become routine and dull. You can become one on a blanket in front of a roaring fire in your fireplace. Making it in the back seat of your car may be exciting for you. For the truly daring, lovemaking can be, both figuratively and literally, a mountaintop experience. The two of you can climb a mountain, make a blanket of your clothes or take a blanket with you, and enjoy each other's bodies. (If you do this, practice discretion and make sure no one else is around.) Tall grass is another good outdoor setting for adventuresome couples, as is a cornfield. I'm sure you get the idea; it is more exciting to make love in an unfamiliar place occasionally than to always do it in your bedroom.

Some couples find it more exciting to have sex where there is a possibility that they will be discovered in the act. If this is true of you, I have a few suggestions to offer to you. First of all, it is important to be fully aware of who might discover you. If it is a stranger, it may not be a big thing for either of you. However, if you are teenagers and you are found by one of your parents, it is a whole different story. A lot of it depends on your circumstances. If you are a married couple, your making love will be acceptable to everyone, except for a few members of the extreme right wing (and possibly the police if you've chosen a place that's so visible that you're violating public decency laws). If you are going to make love in a place where someone may walk in on you, just make sure you have considered all of the ramifications beforehand.

Sex Talk

Permission to be sexual must include freedom to talk openly about our sexuality.

The best lovemaking does not begin in the bedroom, but rather in the verbal interchange between partners. The right comment at the right time can create an atmosphere in which sexual ecstasy will be yours, just as day follows night. You may not be the most poetic person on the face of the earth, but within there is some talent for artistic expression. You don't have to come up with all of the ideas yourself; you can build on the concepts of others. A large part of this type of practice is being alert and open to what life offers you. For example, a couple might be looking out of the window at freshly fallen snow when the woman says, "It's very pretty." her companion replies, "And I'm sharing it with a very pretty woman." Or they're watching a movie in which a man says to the woman, "Your beauty is only exceeded by your wisdom." If the male movie-goer says to his companion, "Your beauty is not exceeded by your wisdom," she is likely to smile and enjoy the comment immensely. Did this mean that she is not wise? NO, it meant that her beauty is very great. You see how by a clever turn of a phrase from another source, one can enhance a relationship. No one is born with this ability to turn a comment into a new and improved compliment; it's learned through practice. You can learn it if you are willing to put forth sufficient effort. Freedom to practice different comments is yours; you can do it in front of a mirror if this will help you.

If you are uncomfortable with attempting to turn phrases into clever comments, it's okay. An alternative is a straight-forward compliment. You can comment favorably upon your partner's clothes, hairdo, jewelry, perfume, etc. Be bold. All women like to be told they are gorgeous. Men like to hear it too, for all of you women reading this.

Many people refrain from giving compliments because they have poor ego boundaries. They are afraid of becoming too vulnerable because they are ego-involved with their opinions. They want the other person to respond favorably and if that doesn't happen, they think they have failed. This is because they don't understand how to give a compliment, and they do it with ego attached. There is a healthier way to do it. When I give a compliment, it is a gift to the other person. Once I have given it, I have no more involvement with what happens. I have done my part and it is up to the other person to do what she or he chooses with it. If you truly give a gift, then once it is accepted, you have no more control over it. If I give a very nice book to a friend, once it passes into his or her hands, I have no more control over it. Should the recipient drop it in the mud or lose it, it is not my problem. Once I have given the gift, the total responsibility for using the gift rests with the person who received it. The same thing is true of compliments. I, of course, have also encountered people who, because of their upbringing, have trouble accepting positive strokes. Some women, for example, find it difficult to accept a compliment such as, "You're gorgeous." But if they're told this a number of times over a period of a month or two, they may learn to receive it graciously.

Your task it to foster mutual giving and caring in your relationship. With this in mind, give sincere compliments to each other. Phony flattery will be seen for what it is by your partner and will detract from your bond.

It is important to understand the difference between flattery and compliments. Flattery is to praise insincerely, effusively, or excessively. On the other hand, a compliment is a sincere expression of praise, commendation, or admiration. Compliments increase the trust between two people while flattery destroys trust. Compliments increase self-esteem. A sincere comment to your partner conveys loving and caring. If you care for someone, you will give them your attention. Attention is one of the things people want the most, particularly in an intimate relationship.

Flattery decreases self-esteem because it is a lie, and both people realize it. One who flatters seeks to control the one whom he or she is flattering. In other words, the person who offers insincere praise has a hidden agenda. Therefore, it is easy to see why flattery is the enemy of intimacy. If you say to your partner, "You are the most beautiful (or handsome) person on earth," it is flattery. On the other hand, if you say, "To me, you are very beautiful (or handsome)," it is a compliment. The first comment is competitive and has more to do with the person who says it than with the one who hears it. Whether the flatterer is trying to manipulate another person or is obsessed with having the most attractive partner on earth, he or she is trying to meet her or his own ego needs and is really not concerned about the other person. In either case, people like this see their partners as objects and are incapable of true intimacy and caring.

SEXUAL SLANG

When I was about ten years old, I was in a boys' Sunday school class with all boys. One Sunday we all got to class before the teacher did. One of my peers decided that he was going to ask the teacher what he called his sex organ. When our teacher appeared, the boy asked the question. Our instructor turned purple, then red, and finally was able to utter the word, "penis." According to him, this was the only name he had for his sex organ. Looking back on this experience, I don't think he was honest with us. Slang names for the penis and vagina have been around for a long time. Some terms for the penis are: cock, pecker, prick, dong, one-eye, meat and rising star. Examples of terms for the vagina include: cunt, pussy, golden triangle, beaver, love canal, pleasure caravan, and the ultimate slide. Some people are offended by such terms. If they offend you, then don't use them. One the other hand, providing you don't find them offensive, they can enhance your sexual expression. To most men it is much more erotic if their partner says, "Your cock feels just right," instead of, "Your penis feels just right."

Many women find it to be sexually stimulating if their partner says, "Your cunt is so hot," rather than "Your vagina is so hot." Vagina is a very unwieldy word, even more so than penis. Using sexual slang is appropriate only when both partners are comfortable with it. If one partner is comfortable with it and the other is not, you can experiment with it. Through a process of experimentation, the one who is uncomfortable with it may become more at ease with the use of this language. However, if your partner remains uncomfortable with sexual slang and does not want you to use it, then you must stop using it if you want to have a healthy relationship. A sound partnership can only be based on mutual respect and it is very important for each partner to respect the viewpoint of the other. Remember, the use of sexual slang is not essential to your love life.

Cᴏɴᴠᴇʀsᴀᴛɪᴏɴ Wʜɪʟᴇ Mᴀᴋɪɴɢ Lᴏᴠᴇ

Couples vary widely in their behaviors in the embrace of passion. If you are fairly new lovers, it is important to find out what pleases your partner. This can be done best by talking about it. Unfortunately, however, many people find it difficult to have open discussion about what pleases them sexually. This results from the shame and guilt that are all too often associated with the subject of sex in the teaching of organized religion. Again this is a distortion of what God intended for us. We were created to have sexual pleasure, and talking about what turns you on is healthy and perfectly acceptable. Of course, excessive chatter during physical intimacy is undesirable because it will likely interfere with the sensual bonding that makes sex between partners who are totally committed to one another so great! Words of love and caring will increase the strength of the bond and enhance the pleasure of intercourse.

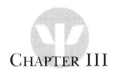

INTIMACY

INTIMACY WITH ONESELF

B efore you can experience intimacy with another person, you must come to know yourself on an intimate level. For that to occur, you must be in touch with your innermost self. If you are a shallow person, this will be very difficult, if not impossible, for you. You want to get in contact with your core values, to be aware of what is most important to you. In this endeavor, you will become aware of what you stand for as a person. It is vitally important that you be completely honest with yourself in this process. If you are not, the results you achieve will be unsatisfactory. The best way to begin to become closer to yourself is to write in a journal. You can write about what is most important to you in your life. It is important to write about feelings when you journal. If you have great difficulty with this task, you may need to seek out a therapist to assist you in getting in touch with who you are.

DIFFERENT TYPES OF INTIMACY

When we consider the issue of intimacy, we must recognize that there are several different levels and ways in which people are close to one another. The areas of close association we will look at include: occupational, intellectual, recreational, esthetic, familial, spiritual, emotional, and sexual intimacy.

Desire for Intimacy

As a psychologist, I have noted a strong desire for intimacy on the part of every client I have worked with. It is also a deep need within myself. We were created to have a very close connection with other human beings. We strive to reach others in this way, but many times it does not work. It is good to come to understand why problems exist, for then we can overcome them. I know of a woman who is afraid of losing her sense of identity in a relationship. As a result, she is always on guard against this threat and intimacy with her is impossible. In order to experience a deep attachment to another person, you must have a strong sense of who you are, otherwise you will be completely overshadowed by the other person. If this happens, you will not be able to have a real closeness because one of you will have disappeared. The desire for intimacy is universal, yet it remains a very rare phenomenon because there are several serious barriers to it in our lives.

Materialism: The Main Barrier

We live in a highly materialistic society. At every turn we are urged to acquire more possessions. We are bombarded daily with messages telling us to we need more and more "things," implying that we are not okay as we are, so we must strive to obtain wholeness through material objects. But it is contrary to my whole life experience to expect to find lasting satisfaction in objects. In fact, the unrelenting pursuit of material wealth often leads to disillusionment and unhappiness.

Materialism is defined as: "Preoccupation with or emphasis on material objects, comforts, and considerations with a disinterest in or a rejection of spiritual, intellectual, or cultural values."[1] In view of this definition, it is easy to see why we have difficulty getting close to one another. If we are disin-

---

[1] Random House Unabridged Dictionary Second Edition. Copyright 1993.

terested in or reject the spiritual and cultural values of another person, we will never understand them.

A materialistic society is inevitably shallow. When we worship at the altar of material goods, we do not understand the advantages of having a spiritual encounter with another human being. We lack an identity beyond our possessions and we are left with a vague feeling of emptiness in the midst of our material wealth. Where the emphasis on the accumulation of "things" is greater, there is often the greatest spiritual poverty and a lack of intimacy. This is no accident; it is a logical development. To obtain, conserve or even to spend great material wealth requires a considerable amount of time and effort. In order to devote sufficient time to this enterprise, a person must neglect her or his spiritual growth. There simply isn't time for both. If you think there is, you're not being honest with yourself.

THE GOD THAT FAILS

Materialism as a god will fail human beings every time. Our society is disintegrating because we lack a common identity and common goals that would take us beyond materialism. The worship of things divides people. If my salvation depends upon acquiring more and more things and you are striving to acquire these same things, then we must be in competition. We cannot be allies or friends, but instead we must be enemies. When material objects are God, it becomes easy to shoot another person for a jacket or a pair of sneakers. The ability to identify with another human being, to achieve intimacy, is gone.

BARRIER II: CONTROL

Another major block to intimacy is the desire to control others. The drive to be in control is particularly strong in men. We are conditioned to make every attempt to control our destiny. In previous generations this macho approach to life was necessary and even an advantage. When settlers moved to the frontier, it was important for men to be strong. They had to contend with many elements and pressures. Males were primarily responsible for providing for their families; they had to provide food and safety. Thus, it was normal for them to make every effort to be strong and to be in control. They probably didn't experience much intimacy with their wives beyond sexual intercourse, but it was not their primary concern. They may even have been unaware that other types of intimacy existed.

Many men exhibit this macho behavior today. They try to portray an image of total self-sufficiency, needing women only on a sometime basis to be of service to them. They may want the "little woman" to cook for them or to be available for sex. These macho men are spiritually dead and will never enjoy deep intimacy in their lives as long as they carry on this charade. When they are seen in therapy, they often break down sobbing as the cracks appear in the false front they have built for themselves. They are also the ones who become desperate if the woman in their life threatens to leave them. They pretend they are dependent on no one; they are in fact very dependent and afraid.

Attempting to control one's wife or partner will preclude achieving intimacy with her. This is equally true when a woman strives to control a man, which is not unheard of. Intimacy can only be achieved between equals. You do not control an equal; you have power only over your inferiors. Oneness with another human being requires a high level of respect, the kind of respect one does not have for an inferior. You cannot treat a partner as if he or she is less important than you are and really bond with him or her.

OCCUPATIONAL INTIMACY

Two people working together on a project may become of one mind and see things in an identical way. There is a thrill in knowing that another human being sees things as you do; there is something life-affirming about this type of experience. The two people may know very little of each other on a personal level, but it doesn't matter because they are not seeking intimacy on any other level. This type of like-mindedness has nothing to do with sex or gender, it can occur between two women, between a man and a woman, or between two men. One of the best examples of this type of intimacy is the following quotation:

> "We are two men, two minute sparks of life; outside is the night and the circle of death. We sit on the edge of it crouching in danger, the grease drips from our hands, in our hearts we are close to one another, and the hour is like the room, flecked over with the lights and shadows of our feelings cast by a quiet fire. What does he know of me or I of him? Formerly we should not have had a single thought in common—now we sit with a goose between us and feel in unison, and are so intimate that we do not even speak." [2]

This illustrates how two people can be very close to one another without knowing much about each other on a personal level. An outside threat in this case, war, tends to unite people and bring them closer together. Food can also bring people closer to one another. In this case, it is the act of sharing a goose, a great treat for them, since they have been existing on army rations. They are soldiers and may be killed tomorrow. This heightens their experience and increases their ability to savor the moment.

[2] ReMarque, Erick Maria. *All Quiet on the Western Front.*

The importance of food as a tool to help establish intimacy between people cannot be overstated. When friends come to our home, we offer them food and drink. Indeed, even when friends bring with them someone you have never met before, you offer this stranger refreshment. This conveys caring and nurturing; by offering these gifts to our friends, we are sustaining their lives. Breaking bread together is actually sharing life with one another.

We Christians have as our model the most intimate meal Christ had with his disciples, the Last Supper. At this event, Jesus shared not just bread and wine, but the very essence of his life. The bread and wine were symbolic of his coming death. He was giving up everything for those whom he loved. We are seldom called upon to give up everything. We are, however, called to care about our fellow human beings.

INTELLECTUAL INTIMACY

There are several types of intimacy, and we may cross from one type to another and two or more areas may easily become intermingled. This is the nature of human interaction and it is healthy and normal.

Closeness on an intellectual level takes place most often in academic settings. When we are able to discern an idea or a concept in the same way as others do, we come together on a common plain. Our ability to have this close association of ideas is not limited to the living; we can have the same experience with people who are dead, through their writings. When we read the work of someone from the past, we get to look into the author's mind and also into the era she or he writes about. We can truly visit the past.

In my work as a psychologist, I achieve an intellectual intimacy with my clients. It is not a closeness between equals, because I know the most private aspects of their lives and they know little or nothing about my personal life. Even so, we are able to reach a rapport rarely seen in other settings. This comes about as a result of the deep trust developed between us. The client must believe in my ability to help him or her. Clients also must sense a deep respect for their personhood on my part. This trust results in a bond of great strength and endurance. Only after it is formed can psychotherapy proceed successfully.

Consider a man who comes to me with the problem of impotence. This is a very personal issue and is very threatening to him for several reasons. First, it relates to his very nature, his functioning as a sexual being. Second, it casts doubt on his sense of masculinity. Third, it makes it very difficult for him to maintain an ongoing relationship with his partner. In this situation the man's greatest fear is that his problem will never be solved. What he receives from me at this time is reassurance concerning his ability to overcome the problem. He is also treated with respect as a human being. If he shared this problem with his friends (especially casual friends), he might well receive ridicule instead of support. (This is a sad commentary on the so-called friendships between men in our society.)

In working with me, he finds an atmosphere of acceptance in which his problem is taken seriously. He learns step by step how to solve the problem.

RECREATIONAL INTIMACY

Play is important for people of all ages. Many adults, however, have lost the ability to play because they are concerned about what others will think of them. They see play as appropriate only for children. By "play" I don't mean organized games such as baseball, softball or volley ball. Instead, I am referring to spontaneous, enjoyable activity engaged in for its own sake. Being able, in this sense, to play with your spouse or partner will strengthen the bond between you. The freedom and willingness to play with your partner can add a whole new dimension to your relationship. This playfulness will most likely carry over into your sex life and help to make it more fun and exciting.

When you have an outdoor adventure together, for example, you will always be able to savor the experience in the future. Being close to nature provides you with an opportunity for spiritual renewal. When you observe God's creation up close, you get a sense of awe and wonder, and this revives your spirit. It doesn't matter what you do as long as you both enjoy it. A hike in the woods near your home may be ideal for you. Many people enjoy walking around a lake. Some people seek more strenuous activity such as bicycling, swimming or running. Strenuous activity has the added benefits of prolonging your live and helping you feel better.

Romance

Engaging in recreational activities together provides you with an excellent opportunity for romance. Romance will fade in your relationship over time and you can accept this with grace and understanding if you are mature. This by no means precludes romantic experiences in your lives. The most treasured memories of many couples are special times they have shared. A spectacular evening can begin with a fire in the fireplace, the right music playing, a glass of your favorite beverage, flowers, poetry, or anything else you want to add. Some people find it to be more romantic to be in a different place with their beloved. Certain natural settings may greatly enhance in your relationship. A visit to one of our national parks such as Yellowstone or Bryce Canyon may be the ticket for you. Certainly going to the grotto in Hawaii and hearing the Hawaiian Wedding Song was a very romantic experience for me. My slogan is: "Enhance through romance." It is common for us to idealize our beloved. Many people are uncomfortable with being idealized; my suggestion is for you to relax and let it happen. And to enjoy it.

Recreation gets you away from your daily routine, and thereby can give you fresh life, restore your strength, and revive you. Engaging in activities with your spouse or partner can give your relationship fresh life, restore its strength, and revive it. There are great moments for us as human beings if we will open ourselves up to them.

AESTHETIC INTIMACY

If you are able to appreciate beauty in your life, then you have been given a real gift. When you are able to share your vision of what you find particularly attractive with your beloved, your relationship will become ever more special. You don't have to see things in exactly the same way. What is a great source of joy is for each of you to listen to the other's description of what is aesthetically appealing.

A way to begin is to explore nature. You can do this in your own neighborhood. God puts on a spectacular show every clear evening with a sunset. Watching this together, hand in hand, in a spirit of peace and tranquillity, has to bring you closer together. You can plant a flower garden together and have the closeness that comes from enjoying the beauty of the blossoms that come forth. Exploring nature will foster spiritual development in your union and allow you to feel the intense joy of being one with the earth. Obviously, the different types of intimacy are not mutually exclusive; rather, they're integrated into the mosaic of life.

There are certain natural sights I recommend highly. I will begin with three: the Grand Canyon, Bryce Canyon and Niagara Falls. Seeing these sights—some of the wonders of the world—is an experience beyond the ordinary. It is high adventure that can provide you and your partner with a lasting feeling of appreciation for what we have available to us in this great land. You may develop a thankful heart, and this thankfulness can easily carry over into your relationship with your lover.

I have ridden down into the Grand Canyon on the back of a mule, floated through it on a raft and stood at the top of the wall and peered into this awesome sculpture crafted by God and the river. At the end of the raft trip, I flew out in a helicopter, straight up the wall. It was an experience I will never forget, and I look forward to sharing it with the woman in my life because she has never seen it. Encountering this scenic wonder makes it easy to place your own life in perspective. You are not the center of the universe, and the Colorado River will be flowing through the canyon long after you are dead. Discovering a sense of humility through an experience like this can deepen your relationship by allowing you to open up, to get beyond an egocentric state.

Likewise, being in Bryce Canyon at sunrise or sunset allows you to see the full glory of nature. Again, this is an experience to enhance your relationship. It will lift your spirits to new heights and make glad your hearts. This great wonder of nature, formed over centuries by the forces of the earth and elements, is there for us to enjoy. Niagara Falls can also instill a sense of awe. The word "awesome" has been overused and cheapened in our society, particularly by younger people, but in its purest sense "awesome" is exactly the right word to describe Niagara Falls. When you observe the great rush of water over the cliff, it moves something within you. If it fails to move you, then you are spiritually dead and you may want to take some action to bring life back into your soul.

In speaking of natural aesthetic wonders, I would be remiss if I did not mention Alaska. The vastness of the place gives an idea of the vastness of God. Seeing Mount McKinley is one of those rare experiences in life which lead one to a greater awareness of what the creation of the earth was like. If you see it, you will never forget it, and seeing it with your beloved gives you a moment to cherish together for the rest of your lives. Another important aspect of aesthetic intimacy is appreciating the beauty in your partner. This can encompass his or her physical appearance, but also takes into account the inner person and values the whole being.

FAMILIAL INTIMACY

Normally we grow up in the context of a family and have unique, formative experiences with other members of the family. We retain memories of special events shared within that framework. As adults we may be separated by physical and emotional distance from our siblings and parents, but this does not change the intimacy we had as children. There are, of course, families in which very little closeness exists. People may live together in the same house, but never really share their lives. If there is little trust and nurturing within the family, members will not bond and they will remain distant from one another.

Other families, claiming they are close, are actually bound together by unhealthy ties. In such situations, there will be the dominant and the dominated. The dominant person controls other people in the family either overtly or subtly. They can never have true intimacy because they do not relate as equals. Also, the dominated person is usually a pleaser who, seldom, if ever stands ups for her or his rights. This person lacks integrity and can never really be emotionally close to the one or ones who dominate her or him.

In families that enjoy genuine closeness, the members are honest with one another. If one person does something hurtful to another, the injured person confronts the perpetrator. The person responsible for causing the pain will make amends and grow from the experience. This type of behavior requires maturity on the part of the people involved. In so far as intimacy requires maturity it is rare, because emotional maturity is rare.

Spiritual Intimacy

Spiritual experience, most people agree, is one of the higher endowments of the human mind. There is a spirit among the people of the earth. When disaster strikes, people will go to the aid of total strangers. There is a kinship beyond the normal everyday ties of human beings, and we can be thankful for its existence. Spiritual development varies widely among individuals, of course. People who have made greater advancement in this area have a mature concern for the welfare of all other human beings. They have no difficulty seeing members of other races, cultures, and countries as fully human. They are concerned not only about human rights in their own country, but in all nations around the world. These individuals see themselves as stewards of the earth and have considerable concern about preserving the environment for coming generations. We are interested in learning and acquiring wisdom. Looking to the wisdom of past generations is one way we increase our knowledge and grow as human beings.

In our striving, we come to see clearly the importance of being of service to others. In the servant role we continue to learn by observing and listening to the people we serve. The spiritually developing person knows the importance of caring for oneself. She or he takes care of their own health and well-being. We remember the words of Jesus in Luke 10:27: "So he answered and said, 'You shall love the lord your God with all your heart, with all your soul, with all your strength, and with all your mind, and your neighbor as yourself.'"[3] We see the importance of balance in our spiritual quest, loving ourselves as much as we love our neighbors. I have known individuals who always place the needs of others ahead of their own needs. Some of these people think of themselves as more holy than anyone else. In my view, they are persons with low self esteem

---

[3] Holy Bible.

who are unhealthy both spiritually and psychologically. Healthy individuals, while deeply committed to serving to others, are able to say no to the requests of other people when they have reached their limit in terms of time and energy.

Our spouse or lover is the person who deserves the best treatment from us. It is this person who merits our best compliments, time, caring, and nurturing. Sadly, many couples nurture each other less after marriage than they did before. They do not understand the dynamics of a relationship or the great potential within one. In order for our spiritual life to continue to flourish, we must continue to nurture it throughout your lives.

Perfectionism is the enemy of intimacy, particularly spiritual intimacy. When we want our spouse to be perfect in every way, we deny ourselves the joy of being human and allowing our partner to be human. Because we do not accept our lover on a human level, we cannot achieve a true bonding with this person. For example, many men want their partners to be physically flawless, to live up to an idealized, fashion-model or playmate image. When the woman is unable to fulfill this fantasy, she is treated as if she is of less value than others. The opposite is the case for couples with real closeness, because they treat each other with a high level of respect for who they are as persons.

If you and I do things for our beloved out of a sense of duty, without really wanting to, it will not bring us closer together. Instead it will create tension and resentment which will drive us apart. On the other hand, when we nurture our partner with a complete feeling of willingness and joy, it promotes growth in our relationship and in us as individuals. When we see ourselves as one, as a bonded pair with a single purpose, then doing something for our lover is really doing something for ourselves. Couples who have reached this level of understanding and maturity in their development have a deep sense of joy and happiness and are truly blessed.

As a psychologist, I am fortunate to have the opportunity to achieve spiritual intimacy with my clients. I am thankful for the many rich experiences I have had with people with whom I have worked. My work has clearly been of service to those persons who have entrusted me with helping them to care for their lives. My efforts have had a significant impact on the lives of numerous people; this I know, and it is a source of lasting joy and satisfaction for me.

Eᴍᴏᴛɪᴏɴᴀʟ Iɴᴛɪᴍᴀᴄʏ

When we contemplate the process of becoming one with our partner, it may seem as if emotional closeness must come before spiritual closeness. Upon further examination, however, we understand how these types of intimacy develop simultaneously. In learning to trust each other on the deepest emotional levels, it is essential for us to see in the other person evidence of a spiritual self. Genuine caring, giving, and nurturing can emerge only from a wellspring of commitment and maturity. It requires maturity to realize the importance of keeping the confidence of our partner. This is particularly true in our society whose people thrive on gossip. In many circles, the way to be popular is to have some juicy story about someone to share with the group.

When we're in an intimate relationship, we do not share information about our partner without discussing it first. This is simply according our lover respect, the same consideration we expect for ourselves. This is an example of loving your neighbor, or partner, as you love yourself.

Men have great difficulty being completely open on an emotional level. In many cases, they don't know how to go about it. This is because men, in their formative years, often are taught to do the exact opposite. Males have been conditioned to compete with other males for the best score on the golf course, the best job, and the most attractive woman. In order to have the best chance of winning, they have been taught to suppress their emotions, because to show any sign of perceived weakness would reduce their chance of being the alpha male. This phenomenon is clearly exemplified by the distortion of the purpose of sports. Sporting events were originally developed for the purpose of physical conditioning and health. Athletes did their best to win, but their whole world did not collapse if they lost. With the great pressure to win in our society, much of the joy has gone out of sports. When a person plays poorly in a sport, she or he is unhappy and sometimes miserable. When did you last hear a man say, after he lost in golf or tennis, "I really enjoyed playing the game?" Such an attitude is unheard of. We expect someone who has lost to feel bad, to experience shame.

When these men enter a relationship with a woman, their emotionally restricted behavior carries over into this situation. They are unable to be emotionally open with a woman because they are emotionally impaired. A man like this has spent years suppressing his emotions; he isn't going to suddenly be able to express them freely. He will be fearful of displaying any sign of weakness around his partner because he may be seen as unmanly or, heaven forbid, a "wimp." Many women are uncomfortable when a man shows deep emotion and encourage the emotional constriction many men practice. In such a relationship, intimacy cannot possibly happen.

Only by having the capacity to accept a wide range of emotions within ourselves can we achieve emotional oneness with another person. When we are able to appreciate the feelings our partner is having in a certain situation, it forms a bond between us that mere words can't fully describe or explain. When two lovers enjoy this extraordinary experience, they are transported to a new height in their life together. If you are among the fortunate few who are able to be free enough emotionally to feel deeply, then your heart is full of gratitude and your life is rich beyond any material wealth. If you are incapable of this type of behavior at the present time, but would like to learn it, there is a questionnaire at the end of this chapter, which will provide you with a place to begin.

Sexual Intimacy

We live in a society where instant gratification and impulsive behavior are portrayed as normal and healthy. This idea is reinforced through our media and entertainment. It is common to see people in movies or on TV meet one another and start sleeping together all in one day. When this attitude pervades the sexual sphere of a person, usually a male, it carries with it an aura of selfishness and precludes the possibility of intimacy. The result is sexual exploitation, or, to put it crudely, fucking, rather than making love. In this scenario the person (usually the male) has no interest in the needs of his partner. He is immature and self-centered with no real capacity for closeness. Actually, he fears deep attachment to a woman because his own identity is unclear and he believes that he may lose himself if he becomes too close to another person. He feels he doesn't have much to offer and he is probably right.

Making love is a very different experience. In the first place, the couple has achieved emotional and spiritual intimacy and there is genuine caring and nurturing in their relationship. They trust each other and feel safe with one another. They are interested in their own pleasure, but also the needs of their partner. It is in such a context that we can be of service to one another. By demonstrating deep caring for your lover, you show love for her or him as God has demonstrated love for you. Thus, you and your beloved communicate on a spiritual level during your lovemaking. When you bring pleasure to your partner through foreplay, loving words, and sexual union, you participate in God's creation, for we were created female and male.

FREEDOM

An essential element in this type of bond is freedom. Both the woman and the man must enter into the sexual encounter of their own free will. Any hint of coercion or manipulation will destroy any chance of gaining a deep emotional bonding. Respect for the personhood of your lover is an essential ingredient for the growth of your relationship. If it is part of your togetherness, you cannot fail; if it is not, you cannot succeed.

Two practices that are significant barriers to intimacy are manipulation and coercion. Women probably manipulate men more often than the opposite. This is because a woman's control of a man must be subtle in order to protect him from being seen as less than masculine, or in popular parlance, a "wimp." She doesn't tell him what to do directly, but when he fails to do what she wants, she may pout and act very hurt. For example, if he fails to bring her flowers when all her friends are getting flowers from their men, he will be in for a miserable day. This type of behavior will never lead to intimacy because the woman has a hidden agenda and the man experiences a lot of confusion trying to figure out what that agenda is. She will use energy keeping him guessing and he will expend effort in trying to understand her. In a healthy interchange, they could both use their energy to become closer and more in touch with each other.

Coercion is also too often a part of the sexual landscape in our society. In my experience, men use coercion more than women. A man may attempt to coerce a woman into having sex with him by threatening to leave her if she refuses. Men also too frequently use force in order to get sex. Obviously, the use of force or coercion will never promote intimacy in a relationship between a man and a woman. Only through mutual consent and agreement can two come together and truly bond to become one.

Sexual intimacy can be the crown jewel of your life together. It is shared and fully known only by the two of you, your unique union. The intensity of your orgasms together and the astounding pleasure they produce will bind you together in a physical, emotional, and spiritual way beyond your full understanding. The ecstasy in your bond will permeate your lives and raise you to great heights in appreciation of the senses and sounds of the entire environment in which you exist.

Requests for Tender, Loving Care

A highly effective way to maximize your bond is to adopt the practice of making special requests. In other words, ask your lover to do something special for you. A massage, a particular meal, a meaningful song, poetry, a trip to a place where you had a very enjoyable time, these are all things to add to the romance between you.

To make this practice even more satisfying, I suggest making an agreement between the two of you that provides for only one of you to make a request at a time. The other person must say yes to the desired activity. The partner who carries out the wishes of her or his lover then gets to ask for something at another time. In this way, during each event, the person who requested it is the center of attention and is receiving nurturing without any obligation to reciprocate at the time.

The freedom from any need to do something for your partner in return for what you are getting allows you to enjoy and savor the experience without the tension or anxiety that might result from thinking about how you are going to please your lover. In addition, this practice teaches us how to receive from others, to accept nurturing and revel in its abundance. I especially recommend it for caretakers who have great difficulty taking from others without giving something in return. These people are under-nurtured and do not realize what it is to be fully human. By allowing themselves to receive tender loving care from their partner, they can grow and for the first time begin to comprehend what God will do for them if they will let go and allow Him to do it.

Intimacy Questionnaire Worksheet

1. How open are you with your lover?
2. Is your partner satisfied with your level of openness?
3. What are you most afraid of?
4. What negative feelings do you have about yourself?
5. What positive feelings do you have about yourself?
6. What are your life goals?
7. What are your feelings toward your father?
8. What are your feelings toward your mother?
9. What events in your life had the greatest impact on you?
10. What are your favorite general fantasies?
11. What is your favorite sexual fantasy?
12. What would you die for?
13. How do you want to be remembered?
14. Are you satisfied with your spiritual life?
15. Who is the most important person in your life? Why?

You may wish to answer these questions on note paper rather than in the book. There are two advantages to doing so.

1. You will have more room for your answers.
2. If someone else, like your partner, reads the same copy of the book, they will not be influenced by your answers.

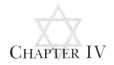

CHAPTER IV

WHAT THE JEWS HAVE TO TEACH US

As I have explored the terrain of human sexuality, one thing has become crystal clear: There are no final answers in this area and there is considerable disagreement as to how we are to live out our lives as sexual beings. Each religious group in our society has its own set of beliefs, attitudes, and teachings about sexual behavior. They provide guidance to their members concerning what is acceptable practice and what is not. Each group believes its belief structure is the correct one according to the Bible, the Koran, or whatever sacred scripture it reveres.

Another part of the picture is a lack of communication and dialogue between various religious traditions in regard to human sexuality. Open discussion would be of benefit to all of us, and one of the purposes of this book is to promote the free exchange of ideas in this area. We can learn from one another and increase our knowledge and wisdom. What issue in human life could be more important? Let us knock down the walls of prejudice and ignorance and walk into the bright light of cooperation!

GUILT AND CONFUSION

I am a practicing Christian and have been raised in the Christian Church. Having observed how the Christian Church traditionally has dealt with sexuality—badly or not at all—I have concluded that there must be something missing; there must be a better way.

49

To broaden my perspectives, I decided to discover what our Jewish brethren had to say on the subject. I spoke with rabbis representing Reformed, Conservative, and Orthodox Judaism. I was very excited about what I learned, and it became clear to me that we Christians can benefit immensely by listening to the Jews. After all, Jesus was a Jew and we come out of the Jewish tradition. I found the Jewish theology concerning sexuality to be positive, spiritual, uplifting, clear, and Biblical, as opposed to the Christian view, which tends to be negative, non-spiritual, guilt-producing, confused, and not necessarily Biblical.

We have been created as sexual beings with the capacity for intense physical pleasure through orgasm. Jews have fully accepted this and are comfortable with it.

THE SABBATH, A DAY OF JOY

One practice, common to all of Judaism, is to encourage married couples to make love on the Sabbath. The Conservative rabbi with whom I spoke went so far as to say he not only encouraged couples to make love on this most holy day, but "commanded" them to do so. "I'm not sure you can 'command' people to have sexual intercourse on a certain day, since it is a personal choice." The Jewish Sabbath is a day of great joy, and Jews are encouraged to celebrate it by engaging in the highly pleasurable act of lovemaking. It is seen as an appropriate way to acknowledge and accept our creation as female and male. Lovemaking is seen as providing both a physical bond between wife and husband and a spiritual union between them. This special way of coming together allows husband and wife to communicate at the deepest level possible.

I have been active in Christian circles all of my life and I have never heard of a member of the clergy advocating love-making on the Sabbath to members of his or her congregation. Within many churches, if a clergyperson were to do so, it would cause an uproar. It might even lead to efforts to remove the pastor from his or her job. That's why Christian clergy are reluctant to take risks in this area.

Sexuality cannot be neutral in a theological context. It will be viewed in one of two ways. It may be seen as a great gift from God to enable us to enjoy intimacy on sexual levels. People who subscribe to this school of thought can be sexual without guilt feelings. They can revel in the exquisite joy as well as the profound mystery of becoming one with another human being. This is the position taken by the Jewish tradition.

From an alternative viewpoint, human sexuality is seen in a negative light, as a barrier to our spiritual growth. This is the view held in too many Christian churches. There is so much discomfort with the issue that is often avoided completely. The attitude has been, "Don't acknowledge it and it will not be a problem." This approach has been and will continue to be ineffective because within these churches young people have continued to reach puberty and have to come to terms with their sexuality. They experiment sexually, in part because of the strength of their drive, and some young girls have become pregnant. Then there is a tortured wringing of hands, as no one knows what to do. Despite such harsh reality, the Church has changed little in the way it deals with our sexual nature. Christian clergy have been less effective than they might have been because they are enveloped in the same cloud of guilt and denial that shrouds the rest of us. I believe an examination of the sources of the shame and guilt surrounding this aspect of our lives would be both edifying and instructive. Taking a good, clear, look at the origins of these ideas, enables us to weigh them and decide whether or not they have total authority and validity for our lives. Through this process we can become more informed and leave behind the yoke of shame with which we have been burdened.

Roots of Guilt

Within the Christian tradition the earliest roots of guilt regarding sexuality lie within the Roman Catholic Church. The teachings and practice of this religious body cast sexuality in a negative, disparaging light, portraying celibacy as more holy than sexual love. It begins with the birth of Jesus Christ, whose mother was the Virgin Mary. Christ, according to Catholic theology, lived out his life as a celibate individual. This is sound teaching because Jesus was, after all, God. He was the only begotten child of God. It was not God's plan for Jesus to father children, who would have been the grandchildren of God. If Jesus had fathered children, it would have been theologically confusing and would have destroyed his mission on earth. Never the less, I believe Jesus was certainly capable of fathering children, for he was a man. He simply chose not to follow this path.

Roman Catholics have sought to further repress sexuality through their teaching about the Virgin Mary. In their belief system, Mary not only was a virgin until the birth of Jesus, but remained a virgin throughout her life. Thus, according to the Catholic Church, two of the most revered figures in Christianity, Jesus and his mother, the Virgin Mary, never engaged in sexual intercourse and remained celibate throughout their lives. This is the foundation for the practice of celibacy of nuns and priests. While I accept the idea of Christ living a celibate life and understand its biblical implication I do not accept the premise that Mary remained a virgin.

In fact, I believe that the Bible directly contradicts this view. In Matthew 1:24, we find "When Joseph awoke, he did as the angel commanded and brought Mary home to be his wife, but she remained a virgin *until* her son was born and Joseph named him Jesus."[4] It says nothing about Mary remaining a virgin for life, only until Christ was born. So Mary remained

---

[4] Holy Bible.

a virgin until the birth of Jesus, and then she became sexually active with her husband Joseph. But engaging in sexual intercourse with her husband in no way diminishes her importance in the Christian story and does not affect her character or holiness. It does not cast her in a negative light. It just allows her to be fully human.

In Mark 3:31-32 we read, "And his mother and his brothers came; and standing outside they sent to him and called him. And a crowd was sitting about him; and they said to him, 'Your mother and your brothers are outside, asking for you.'" Jesus had brothers, and for that to be the case, Mary had to give birth to other children. For that to occur, Mary had to have sexual relations with Joseph and be impregnated by him. Mary was created to be sexual and called to be holy, just as we are. Sexual activity does not detract from Mary's holiness or her role as the mother of Jesus. If it is upsetting to think of Mary as the lover of Joseph, then one might ask if there is something unsavory, indecent, or even sinful about sexual love between a wife and husband. That, I think, the subtle message perceived by many, if not most, members of the Roman Catholic Church. A negative view of human sexuality is always implied in the way the Church venerates celibacy.

A Theory

The sex drive is one of the most powerful forces known to humans, yet the Catholic Church requires that its priests and nuns subjecate their sex drive. They must bring their sexual desires under complete control. They are taught this and are conditioned to follow this practice. Violating their pledge of celibacy is seen as a serious violation of their most sacred vows. In this context some do break the celibacy rule, as we know from several well-publicized cases of priests who have done so. This attests to the strength and power of the sex drive with which people have been created. It also speaks to the sublime pleasure of sexual union, given to us by God as a gift. If a person is going to give up all of this, she or he may well ask what they are going to get in return. The Catholic Church promises them a closer relationship with God than they could have if they become sexually active. If you are going to take away something major like the opportunity for ecstatic pleasure and complete intimacy with a fellow human being, then you had better provide something major in its place, such as a special relationship with God.

Power may also be a factor in the demand for celibacy. If the Church can control the expression of your sexuality, the most basic, fundamental aspect of who you are, it becomes easy to gain control over other areas of your life. I see the insistence on celibacy as unsound from a psychological as well as a theological viewpoint. Further, if we as Christians can accept the sexuality of Mary, the mother of Christ, it will make possible the full appreciation of our own innate sexual nature and the full realization of it with a minimum of guilt.

Judaism regards the sex act as a way to celebrate, to become whole, and to achieve holiness. As lovemaking draws us together, it brings us closer to God. Sexual intercourse is seen as a source of pleasure and a way to participate in procreation.

SPECIFIC PRACTICES

In the Reformed Jewish teachings, masturbation is seen as normal. This idea is conveyed to Jewish youth because they don't want their children to feel bad about their sexuality. According to a Conservative rabbi with whom I spoke, masturbation is seen as a normal sexual activity, so there is no attempt to place any guilt on those who practice it. In the Orthodox circles, however, sexual self-gratification is viewed as being unnatural. It is considered a waste of semen in the case of a male. They see the possibility of sperm being productive, possibly impregnating a female. Therefore they oppose ejaculation where semen is deposited on the ground or in the toilet.

Reformed and Conservative Jews sanction all types of sexual expression as long as there is mutual consent between the partners. Oral-genital sex is not condemned because the act of lovemaking is viewed as a source of pleasure. Sodomy is okay between consenting adults. On the other hand, the Orthodox Jews do not recommend oral-genital sex and come close to forbidding it. They would never approve of sodomy, and they regard it as a crude abomination and a sign of psychopathology. There is clearly a significant difference in the approach to sodomy by the different Jewish traditions.

Orthodox Jews have no formal sex education program. The rabbi with whom I spoke was in favor of developing such a policy. The Reformed and Conservative traditions both have extensive sex education programs. The rabbi from the Reformed tradition does not hesitate to address the issue of sexuality from the pulpit.

HOMOSEXUALITY

Reformed Jews have individuals teaching in their schools who are openly homosexual. They have affirmed the ordination of gays and lesbians, a number of whom serve as rabbis. The rabbi with whom I spoke indicated that there are many members of his congregation who oppose openness towards homosexuals. He did know of one adult male who was married and gay who committed suicide. The reasons for his action were surely complex, but one reason was presumably his inability to come to terms with his homosexuality. The Reformed Jews will be blessing homosexual unions within five years, according to the rabbi. He himself would not have participated in a ceremony of this type three years ago, but would today.

Conservative Jews see everyone as being created in God's image, including homosexuals. They have rabbis who are gay and they receive the same treatment as heterosexual rabbis.

Still, congregations vary in their acceptance of gays and lesbians; some are very accepting and some are quite intolerant. The level of acceptance is heavily influenced by the attitude of the clergy in the particular congregation, of course. The Conservative rabbi with whom I spoke has counseled people who have "come out of the closet." He has been comfortable in this role and has been a source of comfort to those who have sought his guidance in this critical time. He sees homosexuality as an issue that must be addressed. But to him a more important problem is the lack of monogamous relationships. Having multiple relationships, whether they are hetero-, homo-, or bisexual, is perceived as clearly sinful. As we are partners with one God, we are to be partners with one person. Promiscuity runs in direct opposition to this theology. In my view, one who does not practice monogamy destroys her or his chances for achieving intimacy for which we have been created. Such a person will never know the joy, peace, and great sense of well-being available to us until he or she commits to one person.

The Conservative rabbi views the sexual union of husband and wife as being symbolic of the relationship between God and Israel. In this theological system, the way you treat your partner represents how you relate to God. It is easy to discern how important it is to be loving to your spouse in this context. If we all practiced this, there would be a lot more happy marriages than there are currently. If we truly became one with our partner, which is possible, a lot of the conflict we see in relationships would cease.

The rabbi from the Conservative tradition views the Christian doctrine of original sin as a rejection of the body. This presents a difficult dilemma for Christians because the body is where we live. It is important not only to accept your body, but to appreciate it and treasure it. An important aspect of this is to take care of your body—by eating healthy foods, drinking healthy liquids in sufficient quantities, and getting enough exercise. In many ways our culture conspires against all of these things. A plethora of products in our society serve to undermine health, and consuming these products will not only have a negative impact on your physical, mental, and spiritual health, but possibly on your sexual health as well. I refer primarily to alcohol, drugs, and tobacco products, but I will also include junk food and food high in fat and sodium.

Orthodox Jews are the most conservative. The rabbi with whom I spoke was named Barry. According to Barry, we were created sexually for procreation. This is the main reason for sexual intercourse and pleasure is secondary. He did emphasize the sacredness of sexual union, which I have already mentioned elsewhere. Barry addressed the issue of birth control. In the Orthodox tradition, the use of birth control practices by women is approved. A woman may use oral contraceptives or an I.U.D., or may have a tubal ligation. A man, on the other hand, should not use birth control devices, such as condoms. Again, this has to do with the orthodox view of semen, which they believe should always be expended for procreation.

Barry noted the Orthodox approval of scientific methods of achieving pregnancy as long as the sperm of the husband is used. Rabbinic consultation must be part of the process. Sexual union outside of marriage is discouraged. Both women and men expect to marry a virgin.

If a gay person wants to join an Orthodox Synagogue, will pray in an orthodox way, and will behave with dignity, Barry believes the person would be accepted in most congregations. What the person does in private is her or his own business. As long as the person's behavior does not hurt anyone and the individual does not publicly exhibit his homosexuality, it is acceptable. Barry and the other clergy could blind themselves to reality and order gay Jews to be celibate, but they realize how unrealistic that would be. They accept the sexuality of human beings and understand the need for it to be expressed.

In Orthodox Judaism, if a divorced person wants to marry again in the synagogue, the person is required to go through a religious divorce. This process involves counseling, a written document setting forth the reasons for remarriage, and a divorce ceremony, which is private. As a psychologist who is keenly aware of the healing power of ceremonies, I applaud and appreciate the idea of a divorce ceremony. I see it as the best way to bring closure to the end of the relationship.

According to Barry, many parents are too inhibited about their own sexuality to provide adequate sex education to their children. Communication within families on this issue is very poor. Children in trouble in regard to their sexuality would rarely discuss it with their parents and would be even less likely to discuss it with a rabbi, according to Barry. They would most likely talk to peers about it.

One practice common to all of Judaism is the reading of the Song of Songs in the synagogues during Passover. The whole book is read, and the beauty of the writing is thoroughly enjoyed. It is seen as the story of the romance between God and his people. It is a very sensuous document and speaks clearly to our sexual nature. It is an acknowledgment and celebration of our sexuality that is completely missing from most Christian worship services. The sexual repression that is so common and widespread in the Christian approach has underemphasized or ignored this book. Perhaps it is time for this to change. We can learn something from our Jewish friends in this regard.

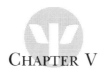

CHAPTER V

WHAT ABOUT HOMOSEXUALITY?

In a discussion of human sexuality, it seems unrealistic to avoid the issue of homosexuality. After all, some people estimate ten percent of the population consists of persons whose primary sexual attraction is to a person of the same sex. This is a sizable group and there are many attitudes toward them in our society.

DISCOMFORT WITH SEXUALITY

There is considerable discomfort with sexuality in general in our culture. The guilt and shame surrounding the central factor of our existence are very unfortunate and are the cause of much human misery. With a pervasive feeling of uneasiness even about heterosexual relationships it is easy to see why some people are extremely upset by homosexual relationships. Homophobia is rampant in the United States; the greatest fear of many parents is that their son or daughter might grow up to be gay.

The sexual identity of many males in our society is very weak. After all, if a man has a strong sexual identity, he will not be threatened by the existence of homosexuals. Because so many males are homophobic and there is so much ignorance about homosexuality, it is a very important subject for me to address.

Bert and Ernie

Within the last few years concerned parents from many parts of the country voiced concerns about Bert and Ernie of *Sesame Street* being homosexual. This contention is absurd for at least two reasons: First of all, Bert and Ernie are puppets and have no sexuality. Secondly, they simply represent two men who have a close relationship and care about each other. Most heterosexual men and women who see this conclude: These two guys really care about each other, therefore they must be homosexuals. After all, two heterosexual men could not care about each other so much.

This explains the loneliness of many so-called "straight" men; they don't dare to get too close to another man or people may think they are gay. This is why so many men are almost totally dependent upon a woman or women for any semblance of an emotional life. These men then become extremely vulnerable in their primary relationships. After all, if your entire emotional support is tied up with your spouse, and she leaves you, it will be devastating. This is why many men will go to almost any length to be re-united with their wife or lover. In my view, it is also one of the main reasons for domestic violence. Men who resort to violence have invested all of their emotional capital with their spouse. Then when the spouse fails to meet all of their emotional needs, they lash out at her.

Returning to Bert and Ernie, if you wonder whether or not exposure to them will turn your child into a homosexual, then what about teddy bears? Does your child sleep with a teddy bear? What is the sex of the teddy bear? If it is the same as the sex of your child, horrors! This illustrates how ridiculous the thinking of some parents can become. With people like them raising children, the future need for psychologists like myself is assured.

WHERE I'M COMING FROM

I am a male heterosexual who has never been sexually attracted to another man. I have had no sexual fantasies about men. Nevertheless, I have close male friends with whom I am able to share my innermost thoughts and emotions. We are free to laugh together and also to cry together. We also hug one another when we want to. I am very thankful for these relationships and believe they enhance my relationships with women and particularly with the woman with whom I have a primary relationship. I am secure in my sexual identity (and I say this not boastfully, but in a thankful spirit). As a result, the lifestyle of homosexuals is not threatening to me. I have gay acquaintances whom I have known for twenty years, and I am able to relate to them comfortably. This enables me to discuss the issue of same-sex erotic relationships in an open, fair and enlightened manner.

A THEORY ABOUT THE ORIGIN OF HOMOSEXUALITY

The natural order of things is sex between a man and a woman. This is how we were created by God. When you consider the physiology of human beings, particularly their sexual organs, you quickly notice how the erect penis slides neatly into the lubricated vagina. This is normal sexual behavior. Since heterosexuals make up 90 percent of the population, heterosexual intercourse is statistically normal, and sexual activity between two persons of the same sex is abnormal. Abnormal is defined as "not normal, average, typical, or usual, deviating from a standard."[5] Homosexual behavior deviates from the standard of sex between a female and a male and is thus abnormal. This conclusion will not please people in the gay community, but I stand by it. I do not believe it is possible to have an open discussion of homosexuality while pretending it is normal.

[5] Random House Unabridged Dictionary Second Edition. Copyright 1993.

Once we agree on the issue of what is normal and what is not, we then need to see where this will lead us. Defining gay behavior as abnormal does not make any moral judgments about it. There are many conditions we define as abnormal. For example, using average intelligence as the norm, both very high and very low intelligence are abnormal. Einstein was abnormal! This is in no way a judgment about the advantages or disadvantages of being abnormal, it is just a statement of fact. So it is with gay sexual behavior; my purpose is to establish a clear picture of how it is seen in the larger context of heterosexual society. When I classify homosexual behavior as abnormal, I am not evaluating it from a moral standpoint; I am only saying it is different.

There is growing evidence that a genetic factor plays role in determining a person's sexual preference. Something seems to happen to the fetus in the uterus to cause a person later to be either heterosexual or homosexual. If this is true, as I believe it to be based on my professional experience with gay people, then its clear that a person has little or no control over her or his sexual orientation. And if this is the case, we have no right to condemn homosexuals. We do not condemn someone who has brown eyes; we should not hate and condemn someone who has a same-sex preference. Those of us who call ourselves Christians, particularly, have an opportunity to love someone who is different from us.

One gay man whom I have known for years talked to me openly about his experience. He indicated how he felt different from other males at a very young age, perhaps 5 or 6. According to him, no one would consciously choose to be homosexual because "no one respects you for who you are." He made clear how difficult it is to feel good about yourself because society at large condemns your life style. There is great hypocrisy in a church that preaches love on the one hand but rejects gays on the other. When he entered his teenage years, my acquaintance denied his homosexuality.

He dated girls for about 5 or 6 years. He was uncomfortable when he acted as if he was a heterosexual, so finally he decided to be what he was. At that moment he experienced integrity for the first time in his life. In other words, he came to himself and accepted who he was, even knowing the price he would pay.

CONSEQUENCES OF ACCEPTANCE

When a person comes to terms with his or her homosexuality, there are numerous factors to be dealt with. For one thing, there is a sense of loss, which can be ongoing. One has to come to terms with the loss of the opportunity for a traditional family. A person will probably never have children. This is a major life shift, since almost all of us grew up in families and expected to have a family of our own someday. A second issue to be faced is the end of the opportunity for a marriage that is recognized by the larger society. In most states, a gay person cannot legally marry a person of the same sex. This may change in the state of Hawaii soon. The losses imposed on homosexuals by their lifestyle can be resolved through a process of mourning similar to the pattern used to resolve grief over any significant loss. I will not delineate the steps here, since they are widely known and practiced in support groups and therapy.

According to my gay colleague, relationships among homosexuals vary a great deal. Some gays are unable to sustain a relationship for a long period of time (just like some heterosexuals). Some are in committed relationships and have been for some time. In other words, homosexuals have the same type of relationship problems as do heterosexuals.

Hereafter I will refer to my gay colleague as John (not his real name) to simplify things. According to John, it is harder for a homosexual to "come out of the closet" later in life because it is harder to find a lasting relationship. In the gay community, according to him, 30 is old. Older members of the group want to take care of younger ones, not unlike so-called "straight" people.

In our discussion, we couldn't avoid confronting the issue of HIV infection and AIDS. According to John, many gays don't care if they get AIDS and die, because they have lost so much through the death of friends and lovers. Also, those who are not HIV infected sometimes feel guilty for being spared when their friends have AIDS and die from it. This phenomenon, called survivors guilt," is common among those who have lived through a situation (e.g. war, concentration camp, earthquake, fire) in which many people around them die. However, there's a significant difference between being afflicted with HIV and being a victim of a natural disaster: In the case of HIV infection, people run the risk of death because of their own irresponsible behavior. In death camps wars, earthquakes, etc., people have no control over their fate. But the experience of guilt for having survived when those around you are dying is the same and speaks eloquently of our human bond, which extends across international borders, generations, and lifestyles.

John would support mandatory HIV testing if there was complete confidentiality concerning the results. Men he has had sexual relationships with have revealed their HIV status before any sexual activity took place. This, of course, is very healthy and is the best way of preventing the spread of HIV, aside from abstinence. When people are first diagnosed as being HIV-positive, they are in shock and may have difficulty telling their partner. If there is sexual activity between them at this point, the infected person is exposing his or her partner to the risk of infection and, as we know, death. John sees denial of the risk of HIV infection as stemming from the overall denial of sexuality in our society. I concur in this view and strive to end the denial of sexuality. Another factor in the lack of disclosure of a person's positive HIV status is the fear of honesty and people's reluctance to be open with one another. It is a barrier to intimacy and a sign of emotional and spiritual immaturity. A spiritually mature person would never place the life of another person in danger, particularly if there was love between the two of them. Such a person would not risk infecting his or her partner with a fatal illness. Anyone who would knowingly risk infecting others has a spiritual disorder and quite possibly a personality disorder.

According to John, even if someone has tested negative for HIV, people don't believe him or her. In fact, simply being tested renders one suspect. This may be a sad commentary on a low level of trust among homosexuals. This would help explain the isolation and loneliness some of them experience.

CONSEQUENCES OF DENIAL

Some individuals remain in denial concerning their true sexual identity for many years, even a lifetime. Some of these people get married and have children. Hiding their true identity from their spouse, they live in deception, an existence without integrity. They pay a high price for their decision, on both a psychological and spiritual level. A person in these circumstances can never experience true intimacy because he or she is not being honest with his or her partner about who he or she is as a human being. A gay person may repress his or her sexual desires for years in an attempt to remain faithful to a spouse. The gay individual will likely become highly dysfunctional in this situation, and the spouse may feel confused, hurt, and rejected. A homosexual in a marriage may begin to have erotic encounters with persons of the same sex. Sometimes the spouse will find out. This discovery can be devastating to the heterosexual person in the marriage. After all, she, and it is usually a woman, has been mislead for years by her husband. The one person in her life to whom she is supposed to be the closest has been something other than what she thought. The gay person has lived a lie and once this is revealed, it is inescapable and irreversible. It is not uncommon for the spouse to wonder if she is responsible for her husband "turning gay." She may have doubts about her sexual attractiveness. She may at first be in denial, believing that her husband only thinks he is gay and somehow he will return to her. She may think that if she makes herself sexier, more alluring, more sexually available, it will bring him back to her. But her best course of action will be to determine if her husband is indeed homosexual. If he is, she will have to make some decisions. Some couples stay together in sexless marriages. In these arrangements, the man usually has a gay lover or lovers and the woman is sexually abstinent. There is no true intimacy in a marriage with this type of arrangement and I would never recommend it. The most common result of the homosexual coming "out of the closet" is divorce.

In some cases, when the gay individual begins to act out sexually with other men or women, he or she may develop a lot of guilt feelings for deceiving his spouse. He may seek out support groups and find support for telling his spouse the truth. In these circumstances it is better for him to tell his spouse the truth rather than to leave her to find out some other way. It will still be an emotional jolt, but it will be softened slightly because it comes directly from the gay individual. In other words, the homosexual had enough respect for his spouse to tell her directly.

If the sex life of the couple has been dysfunctional, which is likely, then learning about her spouse's sexual orientation can help the straight spouse understand why. In the case of a gay husband, the wife now realizes the lousy sex life she had with her husband is not her fault. This can be a great relief to her.

Women may wish to consider their own reasons for supporting the rights of homosexuals. Given the current climate in our society, it is still difficult for gays to be open about their sexual orientation. If a woman contributes to the oppression of homosexuals there is a consequence for her actions. Such oppression will result in more homosexuals remaining in denial of who they really are. A number of them will get married and try to convince everyone, including themselves, they are heterosexual. The homophobic woman or her daughter may be the person who marries a man like this. If he remains closeted, but has sexual relationships with other men, she runs the risk of contracting HIV. If he tells her the truth about his sexual orientation, she will face the trauma of the breakdown of the relationship and possible divorce. The way to avoid these likely pitfalls is to work toward an acceptance of all people in our society no matter what their sexual orientation may be. As societal conditions improve for gays, they will have less and less reason to enter into heterosexual marriages.

MARRIAGE

Marriage is defined as "the social institution under which a man and a woman establish their decision to live as husband and wife by legal commitments, religious ceremonies."[6] As a culture, we have a large stake in marriage. It contributes to stability and order. It is public and a matter of legal record in our country. When a person is married, others (if they are mature and responsible) recognize that he or she is not available as a potential partner. One of the core expectations in a marriage is sexual fidelity. When a couple weds, the ceremony almost always includes a public pledge of sexual faithfulness to each other for as long as both people will live. There are several reasons for a married couple to remain sexually loyal to one another. First, true intimacy can only be nurtured in a loving, caring, relationship in which total trust exists. Sexual faithfulness is required if trust is to be a part of the relationship. Second, a man and a woman, through the

---

[6] Random House Unabridged Dictionary Second Edition. Copyright 1993.

gift of sexual union, are able to have children. They are able to become co-creators with God of another human being. Experience and scientific study have demonstrated the importance of both parents in the raising of these human beings. Parenthood is a very important function in our society. Because of this, we have given major legal advantages to individuals who marry.

In past generations it was common for the woman to be the homemaker and the man to be the one who earned the family income. The man's compensation package usually included health insurance. Many times he paid nothing out of his salary for this coverage. When a woman married a man who had health insurance, she was covered under this insurance, and this is still true today. I refer to the past because today many families have two people earning the family income, and both wife and husband may have their own health insurance. Returning to the past, the wife became eligible for the vital benefit of health insurance simply by marrying her husband. She didn't have any connection to the company he worked for; her existence was of no direct benefit to the company, yet she was given full medical coverage just because she married an employee of the company. Also, any children this wife and husband had were given medical coverage from their birth until they reached adulthood. Sometimes there was a small charge for dependent coverage which was deducted from the salary of the husband, but in other cases the employer paid the entire cost of the family's insurance. The effect of this benefit was to encourage men to marry and to beget children. After all, if a man had to pay all of the medical expenses of his wife and children out of his own pocket, many men would have been unable to afford to get married and probably would have remained single.

Providing health insurance to families has removed a financial obstacle that might otherwise discourage married couples from having children. This is important to our society, because we obviously cannot continue unless there are succeeding generations.

Perhaps the single most beneficial result of marriage is the status it gives a person. It announces to the world the care each partner receives in a special relationship. The partnership in marriage is unlike any other; it has greater potential to meet the most important needs of humans than any other arrangement imaginable.

There is another definition of marriage in the Random House dictionary: "A relationship in which two people have pledged themselves to each other in the manner of a husband and wife without legal sanction—homosexual marriage." Gays want not only the pledge, but also the legal sanction. They want this for a number of reasons. First of all, until their unions are legally recognized, they will never have equal footing with heterosexuals. Without this equality, they will never feel whole. Second, without legal authority, a gay person cannot make medical or other important decisions for her or his partner. In fact, in cases where one person is critically ill and visitation is restricted to family members, the patient's gay partner cannot visit. Legal union would change this and is a major reason gays want to be able to marry.

THE FUNDAMENTAL QUESTION

We are facing a profound questions here: What is marriage? I grew up on a farm in South Dakota. Most of the adults I came in contact with were married. These marriages all involved a man and a woman, individuals of the opposite sex. This has been my bedrock definition of marriage since my birth. Contemplating marriage between people of the same sex is totally foreign to me. In order to accommodate this concept, I must expand my consciousness and my spirituality. Frankly, for me it would be more palatable if a legal union between two members of the same sex were to be called something other than marriage. This would distinguish it from heterosexual marriage, which is a different relationship. I suggest the term "life union" for homosexual partners. This would give gays recognition in society at large and they would enjoy legal rights in regard to their partner. But they would not be married in the traditional sense and their union would not threaten the institution of marriage.

Many people oppose giving any sanction to homosexual relationships because of irrational fears and homophobia. Yet the same people advocate sexual fidelity and an end to promiscuity. Recognition of gay relationships as permanent would possibly bring about more faithfulness in homosexual relationships and thus less promiscuity. Will it mean an end to multiple sex partners for all homosexuals? Of course not; I'm not so naive so as to believe this is a panacea. After all, heterosexual marriage has certainly not resulted in an end to all extra-marital sex. Numerous studies have confirmed the presence of infidelity in "straight" relationships. This is not a behavior pattern unique to homosexuals. But acceptance of gay relationships as legal would likely reduce the level of promiscuity in this sub-culture. If it did, it would save lives, as it would reduce the spread of AIDS. This seems like a worthy goal if we truly love our fellow human beings.

Homosexuality and Salvation

The purpose of human existence is to work out our relationship to God and to find salvation. This belief is held by many people worldwide. This process involves seeking to understand the will of the Holy Spirit and to live one's life as an unfolding of this will in our interactions with other people. We live and strive to do what is right and attempt to avoid what is wrong. Certain behaviors are defined as just, and we believe God approves of them. One example is bearing one another's burdens. When we enter into communion with a fellow human being, say a person who has experienced a death in the family, we have emotional intimacy with that person. The individual is no longer isolated with her or his pain, but becomes a part of a community. This gives strength to the grieving person and enables him or her to bear the loss in the context of love from those who care.

Another goal of most religions is to teach humans what is evil and to instruct them to avoid these things. If one persists in the practice of evil deeds, the consequence will ultimately be the loss of salvation, separation from God, and spending eternity in hell.

Religious conservatives, or the "religious right" as they are called, have a very definite position on homosexuality. They see sexual behavior between gays as evil and they believe those who engage in these behaviors will go to hell. They are perfectly willing to act as if they are God and see those who disagree with them as evil and on their way to hell. These people advocate sexual abstinence for homosexuals, for they see this as the only way gays can obtain salvation. Those on the "religious right" seem to have very little consideration for homosexuals as individuals. They do not concern themselves with whether or not it is realistic to expect homosexuals to abstain from same-sex sexual activity for the rest of their lives. They seem to have no regard for the human needs of gays and apparently are only interested in demanding adherence to their own rigid belief system. This negative approach is one reason for gays' alienation from mainstream religious groups in our society. This condemnation of homosexuality has also contributed to the difficulties gays have encountered in attempting to come to terms, in a healthy way, with their sexual orientation. After all, if religious groups see our core identity as sinful and evil, it is difficult to achieve and maintain a positive self image.

Some religious organizations have had the courage to approach the issue with a refreshing openness. They have been able to consider sexual orientation in the light of the Bible instead of in the darkness of strong emotions and prejudice. These groups include the Evangelical Lutheran Church in America, and the Conservative and Reformed Jewish Traditions. All of these denominations see sexual orientation as something over which a person does not have voluntary control. They advocate accepting gays in worship settings as equals with heterosexuals. Even more important, they support movement toward the day when homosexual couples will receive the official blessing of their particular religious group. These groups also see the issue of sexual abstinence for gays as an unrealistic goal. One can even question whether asking gays to be sexually abstinent is really demonstrating to them the love of God. What it comes down to is whether or not we believe homosexuals really love each other. We were created as human beings with a strong sex drive, and through sexual union we most clearly express our love. Therefore, if gays truly love one another, they will express this love through sexual behavior.

This is not a simple issue, because it is rooted in the complexities of human behavior. However, a number of things are abundantly clear. First, we are created as sexual beings and much of our behavior is influenced by our sexuality. Second, we as human beings are capable of love. No other creatures are so blessed with this ability to form intimate relationships and experience the great joy of becoming one flesh. The normal, healthy, ecstatic, expression of love is through our sexuality. The great pleasure of orgasm bonds us together like nothing else.

All this applies to people whether they are heterosexual or homosexual. If some people are gay through genetic factors over which they have no control, and if they are capable of love, it is normal for them to express this love sexually. I do not believe in a God who would create people with the genetic code of a gay person with a strong sex drive and then condemn these people to hell for acting out their love through sexual expression. Such a God would be unjust and unloving. God is above all else, loving and just. In the end, I do not seek to determine the salvation of those humans who happen to be homosexual. I will leave that decision up to God, where it rightly rests, no matter what humans will say about it.

CHAPTER VI

WHAT THE CLERGY SAY

I n writing about the interrelationship of sexuality and spirituality it seemed appropriate to see what various members of the clergy had to say about this important part of human life. I spoke with a number of pastors, both Protestant and Catholic, and now share with you what they told me.

I spoke with Nick, a black minister who is Protestant. Nick refers to sexuality in his sermons. He advocates sexual abstinence until marriage. He is careful about what he says from the pulpit about sexual behavior. He sometimes counsels married couples who have questions about acceptable sexual practices. According to Nick, the main purpose of sexual behavior is procreation. He also sees it as a vehicle for the expression of intimate feelings between two people, something human beings ought to enjoy. Nick thinks there tends to be a lot of selfishness on the part of men when they have sex. As long as he has an orgasm, the man will be satisfied and not have much concern about whether or not his female partner has a satisfying climax also. Interestingly, in the Reformed and Conservative Jewish traditions, it is considered desirable for the woman to have an orgasm first. This can only occur if the man is concerned about her needs and makes every effort to satisfy her desires. When the woman is first to experience a climax, she becomes much more open to sexual intercourse. The experience of her orgasm results in a great feeling of closeness and euphoria between the couple. If a man truly loves a woman in a mature way, he will naturally be concerned about her pleasure in the sexual act. Again, the Jews are right on target in this regard.

Another Protestant minister I spoke with, Doug, is a white man serving an inner-city congregation. The membership of his church is about 85% black. According to Doug, sexuality comes up regularly in adult Bible study and in youth groups. In his view, the only appropriate place for sexual intercourse to take place is within marriage. Sex outside of marriage is always a sin. Within marriage, he approves of any sexual practice, as long as both partners consent to it. Thus, while he is conservative in saying any sexual intercourse outside of marriage is sinful, he is liberal when it comes to the sex practices of a couple within marriage, where anything goes.

Doug is aware that young girls in his community are often pressured to engage in sexual intercourse by young boys. It is a status symbol for a boy to impregnate a girl. Doug says this status issue is much more important to young black men than it is to whites. It is a sad commentary on the life of these young black people. When the best way for them to obtain respect from their peers is for them to become fathers of children they are incapable of caring for, there has to be a better way. We have a responsibility as a society to show these youngsters a better method of using their energy. Black adult leaders have a particularly strong role to play here, and they can best begin by being responsible in their own sexual behavior.

Doug has done pre-marital counseling and has counseled couples where one of the partners has committed adultery. He sees value in being much more open about sexuality within the church. He has had parents come to him with requests to talk with their children about sexual behavior. He sees the purposes of sexuality as procreation and pleasure. Doug sees kissing and petting as normal expressions of sexuality within dating. Couples must, however, stop short of "going all the way," in his view.

HOMOSEXUALITY

Doug's first thought about homosexual behavior was to characterize it as a sin. He quoted Romans 1:26-27: "Because of this, God gave them over to shameful lusts. Even their women exchanged natural relations for unnatural ones. In the same way the men also abandoned natural relations with women and were inflamed with lust for one another. Men committed indecent acts with other men, and received in themselves the due penalty for their perversion."[7] In his opinion, same-sex erotic relationships are more clearly sinful if people are behaving in this way as a clear matter of choice. The possibility that there is a genetic, predisposition to homosexual behavior has occurred to Doug. After all, he reads and listens to news programs. If there is a genetic predisposition to being attracted erotically to members of the same sex, then it may not be sinful, in his thinking. In other words, if it is an inborn behavior, those affected cannot be held morally responsible for it. If homosexuality is genetically determined, Doug views this as a result of the common condition of humans being sinful. Gays and lesbians are not different because they themselves are particularly sinful, but this is one of many human conditions brought about by the overall state of sinfulness among human beings. I agree with this view.

Incidentally, I want to address the word "perversion," since it was used in the verses quoted from Romans above. It is defined as "any of various means of obtaining sexual gratification that are generally regarded as being abnormal."[8] In my chapter on homosexuality, I defined this type of sexual expression as abnormal. If one seeks sexual pleasure in this way, it is abnormal. What is normal is the sexual activity between a man and a woman. But again, if a person's constitution causes her

---

7 Holy Bible.

8 Random House Unabridged Dictionary Second Edition. Copyright 1993.

or him to be sexually drawn to a person of the same sex, this is not a sinful act, even though it may be abnormal.

I want to return to some comments Nick, the black pastor, made which I believe are profound and worthy of consideration. Nick struggles with the issue of homosexual behavior. He is unsure whether this behavior is sinful. He has difficulty with it, because he sees it as a denial of our creatureliness. After all, we were created female and male with the ability to have sexual relations with one another. The male and female sex organs were designed to fit together. According to Nick, homosexual practice places humans in the position of arbitrarily deciding how they should behave sexually. He does not believe people are born gay and recommends therapy for homosexuals in order for them to become heterosexuals. (I must point out that the experience of my colleagues in both psychiatry and psychology, as well as my own experience, finds no basis in fact for the belief that homosexuality is a choice that can be altered. In other words, the great majority of homosexuals will not be able to change their basic sexual identity, even with extensive therapy.)

I talked with a priest I will call Father Solomon. (It's not his real name, but it has a nice ring to it. Any priest or minister with this name would command instant respect.) Father Sol, as I will call him for the sake of brevity, sees the normal practice of sexuality as intercourse between a man and a woman. The main purposes of sexual behavior are expressing love and procreation. Sol specifically mentioned the expression of love first, which slightly surprised me, since I have always heard the great emphasis the Catholic Church places on procreation.

Sol's pastoral approach is to approve anything two consenting adults want to do sexually in private. The church teaches that sex outside of marriage is always sinful. However, if people are not aware of this doctrine and have sex without being married, they are not guilty of sin.

Sol sees a small number of church members who come to him with questions about acceptable sexual practices especially oral sex. Generally, people over 45 are not having oral-genital sex, but the people who have the most guilt about this activity are women over 45. Many young people engage in this behavior and have much less guilt about it, in Sol's experience. Today, most young Catholic couples live together and have sexual relations before they get married, according to Sol. He attributes the phenomenon to the drive for immediate gratification in our society. The adage, "If it feels good, do it," applies to sexual behavior, since it feels good. Pleasure seems to be the main goal of people in our society, and Sol does not view this as positive. He would like decisions to be guided by a moral structure and not just by the desire for pleasure. I am in his corner in this case.

Roman Catholic schools offer sex education in grades one through eight. (I cannot comment on the quality of the materials since I have not seen them.) In Sol's parish they have an adult forum once a year on human sexuality. This is a move in the right direction, but perhaps the frequency of these sessions could be increased. In the past, mortal and venial sins were all listed in a book in the Catholic Church. This is no longer true, according to Sol, and the definition of sin now depends more on individual conscience. The role of the church is to foster and develop individual consciences in its members. Sol preaches the morality of social consciousness from the pulpit, not specifically sexual morality. Previously, the predominant emphasis of moral teaching focused on sexual behavior, but now it has been expanded to include numerous social issues such as war and peace, homelessness, and how we treat one another in our business dealings. Sol's parishioners have difficulty seeing these as moral issues and are more comfortable limiting notions of morality to sexual behavior. They find it difficult to grasp the concept of making decisions in a moral context in which what is just may be hard to decide. They prefer to limit their moral choices to the area of sexuality, where questions of right and wrong seem much easier to answer.

In Sol's view, it's not a priests job to judge the morality of other people, but rather to challenge Church members to think about how they act. This leads us to a consideration of homosexual behavior. Sol believes in the old saying, "Love the sinner but hate the sin." The problem I have with this approach is there is a tendency for the "hate the sin" outlook to easily become generalized to the person, or sinner, especially for people with poor boundaries. Active gay sexual behavior is not approved, according to Sol. He has heard confessions of homosexual behavior from members of his church. When he sees people who are involved in this type of behavior, he asks them how they got into it and what their intention is for the future. In other words, do they plan to engage in homosexual behavior on an ongoing basis or do they plan to cease this activity. Sol views continuing homosexual practice as something which must be "worked on." He sees a great deal of confusion among church members regarding sexual morality. Sol personally knows of a high school student who committed suicide because he though he was gay and couldn't cope with it. This is a very sad tale in many ways. No doubt the death of this young person brought great pain to his family, who are left with many unanswered questions. His must have been a very lonely death, feeling cut off from all humanity. It raises a fundamental question within our synagogues and churches about our mission and our faith. The question is whether we have any comfort or caring to offer to homosexual individuals. We have to look at ourselves and decide if our houses of worship are big enough for all human beings to come together and experience the presence of God.

THE FEMALE VIEWPOINT

I spoke with a Lutheran pastor whom I will call Ruth. She teaches confirmation classes and has contact with teenagers, some of whom have come to her with many questions about sexuality. She has been asked, whether pre-marital sex is right or wrong. Young adults with sexual orientation concerns have approached her. She sees a real need for sex education and has an approach in mind. In Ruth's view, school teachers should teach the anatomy and function of sexual behavior, or how babies come to be. Then clergy should teach the ethics of sexuality and parents should be involved in teaching values in this area. According to Ruth, however, Lutheran clergy are very poorly equipped to teach about sexuality. First of all, there is no good curriculum within the Lutheran Church. Secondly, many clergy persons have been raised in a context of having many guilt feelings about their sexual nature and are embarrassed by the subject. (Perhaps we Lutherans could borrow from the curriculums of our Catholic and Jewish friends.) Ruth sees parents as even more poorly prepared than clergy to teach their children about sexuality. There have been no discussion groups within her church for adults on sexuality, but she is aware of a need for them. In the current climate, peers are the main source of information about sexuality for teenagers. This just about guarantees that a lot of mis-information about sexuality will spread by teenagers, which tends to perpetuate the confusion about this issue.

Ruth sees two purposes for sexuality: procreation, and having pleasure in a relationship. She sanctions oral-genital sex within marriage as long as both partners are comfortable with it. If one spouse is guilt-plagued about it, it is best if they not engage in it. After all, the expression of our sexual nature should be free and joyful, and if guilt crowds the freedom and joy out, then the fundamental purpose of our intimate encounter has been lost. Ruth cannot, on the basis of scripture, prove sodomy to be a sin between consenting adults. She does not think the church is ready to approve of homosexual relationships. She herself would be comfortable marrying a gay or lesbian couple in a park, but not in her church.

In her work, Ruth encountered a 15-year-old female who'd had a sexual relationship with a girl about her age. This young person was suicidal and came to Ruth with serious, deep questions. One of her questions was "Who am I in God's eyes?" Another was, "Is my behavior deeply condemned by God?" You can see how fundamental these questions are when we consider the issue of same-sex relationships in a theological context. This girl considered suicide to spare her family from dealing with "this mess." If she killed herself, she thought, her parents wouldn't have to be embarrassed about her and her siblings needn't know about her sexual practices. Fortunately, by working with her, Ruth was able to help this girl accept herself and go on living.

A Theory of Some Suicides

Ruth's experience brought to light a theory of mine concerning mysterious suicides in conservative, highly religious families. There have been numerous cases in which a young person is part of what appears to be a fairly healthy family with a solid religious base, and still the youth kills himself or herself. In some cases, these youths take the lives of other family members before ending their own lives. When these tragedies occur, the survivors are totally shocked and mystified by the behavior of their own child. They do not have a clue as to why it happened. I believe it has to do with the sexual desires of the young person. Consider the situation and you will see what I mean. The parents are conservative, religious people with no understanding of or tolerance for homosexual behavior. The child of this couple has been fighting off an attraction to members of the same sex for some time. Finally, the day dawns when the young gay person can no longer deny her or his sexual nature. The young person may attach great importance to being accepted by his or her parents; indeed, this acceptance may be more important than life itself. If the young person perceives her or his parents as unable to understand and accept his or her sexual orientation, it brings about a crisis. The teenager or young adult may fear the loss of the parents' love. At the very least, the parents will have to confront "this mess," as will the person's siblings. To the young person confronting the issues, it may seem to be a lot easier for everyone if he or she just commits suicide. Unfortunately, it isn't easier and may leave survivors in a haunted state where they will remain for the rest of their lives. In addition, it never gives the family a chance to come together and learn to really love the gay or lesbian member.

Killing oneself is a total denial of God's mercy and is, in the end, a cowardly act. Suicide is final, and the wounds it leaves are permanent. It is the end of all possible growth as a human being for the person who dies. There is always a better alternative if the person will seek it. There is also a great deal of support available to a person who is coming to terms with being homosexual. One is only alone in this struggle if one chooses to be alone.

DIVERSITY AMONG PRIESTS

I spoke with another Roman Catholic priest whom I will call Father Benedict, or Ben for short. According to Ben, the Church has coursework in sexuality that is presented to young people in junior high school. It deals with the biology of sex and encourages abstinence until marriage. Officially, the church opposes masturbation and classifies it as an evil act. In other words, the Catholic Church does not approve of any sexual outlet for teenagers. It teaches them to abstain from sexual intercourse until marriage while at the same time condemning them if they dare to masturbate. Personally, Ben does not see masturbation as evil. I echo his view and recognize the need for some sexual outlet for young people. Certainly masturbation is preferable to sexual intercourse in terms of avoiding the risk of unwanted pregnancies. In addition, it avoids the damage done to the self esteem of one who is "dumped" by his or her sex partner and realizes she or he was only being used as a source of pleasure.

Ben sees modern society as being very concerned about sexuality. He speaks about it from the pulpit, but not often. Jesus talked very little about sexuality, according to Ben, so he doesn't see a need to preach about it frequently. The church only approves the missionary position in sexual relations, he says. Most members, Ben notes, ignore the church's strictures in this regard. People should function according to their own inner integrity and conscience with respect to sexual practices, in Ben's view. Pastoral theology tries to help people reach a good-conscience solution to their questions about different positions for sexual relations. Likewise, the solution for homosexuals is to maintain a good-conscience monogamous relationship, just as heterosexuals are taught to do. The church does not view practicing gays as unable to attain salvation. In other words, in Ben's view, the Church is not ready to condemn them to hell.

History

In the past, the Catholic Church saw lesbians and gays as a destabilizing influence in regard to the heterosexual family. Homosexuality was seen as a grave moral disorder. According to Ben, the new catechism is more understanding of lesbians and gays. Ben believes they should be active in the sacraments and not be rejected by the church. He does not believe in the dictum, "hate the sin, love the sinner." Ben has been involved in situations where a homosexual committed suicide because he was unable to see the path to self-acceptance clearly enough. Having gone through this experience, he preaches forgiveness, love and compassion. He welcomes people into his parish regardless of their sexual orientation.

THEOLOGICAL POLITICS

Churches are interested in maintaining themselves, and they fear anything that might break the established order, according to Ben. Therefore, one would expect the churches to have great difficulty coming to terms with homosexuality, and this is indeed the case. Gays and lesbians break the established order and seem to confound many theologians. It is perplexing for the church to know what to do with these people.

According to Ben, the Catholic Church has always seen those who are celibate as having a higher calling than those who are sexually active, even within a marriage blessed by the church. There you have it in black and white, confirmed by a priest ordained in the church. In this view, Catholics who marry and engage in sexual relations can never be on the same level in the Kingdom of God as those who are celibate. Carrying this reasoning a step further, Protestant clergy who are married can never be as holy as nuns and priests who are celibate. When you examine this idea, there is no mystery about why Catholics who are sexually active are uncomfortable with their sexual behavior and some are plagued with guilt about it. In many cases, this guilt prevents real intimacy with one's partner and can be particularly troublesome to those individuals who have a strong sex drive and are highly orgasmic.

A SECOND FEMALE VIEWPOINT

I spoke with a female pastor who was also Lutheran. She was well-qualified to comment on sexuality because she has counseled people extensively in regard to different sexual issues. I will call her Judy. Judy has counseled women who have been raped. She has brought her healing presence to these women, who I'm sure have benefited from their involvement with her. As a female pastor she sees herself being in a bind because, in our society, women have been viewed as bodies, as sex objects much more than men have. Even as a pastor, Judy is sometimes seen first as a woman. As a result, she has had to exercise caution and restraint in counseling males.

Sexuality is not addressed in confirmation in the Lutheran Church, although there are exceptions to this within individual congregations. Judy sees a need for sex education to be part of a continuing process beginning with children at ages 4 and 5. She encounters a lot of confusion about sexuality among church members. People have great difficulty talking about sex, and parents generally are not providing their children with adequate sex education.

Judy has counseled a number of young people who were exploring their sexuality. She has seen several young men who were not clear about their sexual orientation. These men were primarily homosexual. With Judy's support, each of them eventually was able to talk to his family about this issue. The results, as one might expect, were mixed.

Judy approves of oral-genital sex between adults as long as both consent to engage in this type of lovemaking. She emphasized the importance of free consent on the part of each person and I am in complete and total agreement with her about need for full consent from both parties. In Judy's view, sodomy is acceptable as part of the sexual expression between adults if it is respectful and enhances the relationship. Again, there must be full agreement on the part of both partners to enter into this behavior. If there isn't, they should not engage in it. Judy is ready to welcome homosexuals into the church without placing any restrictions on their sexual activity. She would not require them to be sexually abstinent, but would accept them into the worship setting in the context of their being gay or lesbian lovers.

In my conversations with members of the clergy, I found them all to be sincere and well-meaning. There were many viewpoints expressed on various theological issues. I can see great value in dialogue among clergy about sexuality. No one has the whole truth, so by opening up to the ideas of other traditions, all can benefit.

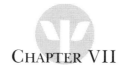

CHAPTER VII

CELEBRATE YOUR SEXUALITY

W e have been created as whole beings, body, mind and spirit. We function best when our actions arise out of the fullness of our existence. In order for our actions to be positive, constructive, yes even holy, we must view ourselves as holy. Generally, we have few problems seeing our spirits as holy. Almost everyone believes in a spiritual existence, even if it not the traditional Christian viewpoint. We also find it natural to celebrate our spirituality and rejoice in the existence of God as spirit. We often feel a oneness of spirit with our fellow human beings when all of us are striving for a common goal. This experience causes us to feel a sense of community with other humans. It is fairly easy for us to attain an awareness of intellectual and spiritual connectedness to other people.

THE BODY OF CHRIST

We hear the church being referred to as the Body of Christ. This concept becomes difficult to grasp because we are alienated from our bodies. This is particularly true of men. In the traditional view, woman is seen as body and man as mind. After all, it is the woman who gives birth. She is also the one who menstruates. Her bodily functions are vital to the reproduction of the species. Also, many men, in their insecurity, would like to keep women focused on the functions of the body so men can handle the important things such as planning, decision-making, and wielding power. Women in our society are conditioned to give a lot of thought to their dress and make-up. This is one way for men to control women. If women spend a great deal of time picking out exactly the right clothes, selecting just the right shade of lipstick, and choosing the best color eye shadow, they will have much less time available to engage in more intellectual pursuits. Keeping women pre-occupied with their appearance gives them less time to be involved in what have been traditionally male functions.

With all of this emphasis on appearance one may ask whether women are more satisfied with their bodies than men are. The answer is a resounding NO! Women have much greater dissatisfaction with their bodies than men do. It is important to look at the reasons for this phenomenon.

Logical Explanation

Advertising begins from a negative premise: "To begin with, there is something wrong with you." Its aim is to convince you of your shortcomings. Because of the spiritual vacuum in our society, this approach is very successful. Once you have accepted this premise, the next step is easy. In order to correct your deficits, you need to buy our product. Your life will become better, people will respect you, you will be somebody. The not so subtly implied message is, "When you own this product you will be happy." We are portrayed as incomplete persons whose lives will be empty until we obtain these items.

This is what marketers tell us day in and day out. Now look more closely at the advertising aimed at women. Much of it revolves around physical appearances. They are continually bombarded with products to improve their attractiveness. Somehow, they are told, they just don't measure up the way they are. Change is required—a new hairdo, new clothes, fake fingernails, you name it and it's out there. In these circumstances, women can easily become discouraged and, feeling they will never attain the ideal body image, give up.

Frustration may lead to compulsive behaviors such as overeating, excessive consumption of alcohol, smoking, eating junk food, or other destructive habits.

When thinking about your body, you may view yourself as part of the Body of Christ. You can also behold your physical self as given to you by God. This is the place you live, it is the way you were created. How you are viewed by society is largely irrelevant to your spiritual development. In order to grow spiritually, it is necessary for you to accept yourself as you are. In accepting yourself, you can still strive to improve. It is important to take care of yourself. It is wise to exercise regularly, eat a healthy diet, get enough rest, and avoid stress-producing situations as much as possible.

SPLIT HUMAN BEINGS

As I said before, we are alienated from our bodies. This is particularly true of men. The practice of functioning primarily on a cerebral plain has become common for men in modern times. We ignore our health and push things to the limit. In past generations, males proved their manhood by performing physical labor and being physically strong. In our current society, the great majority of men work in jobs where intelligence is much more important than muscle strength. In this type of environment, the only avenue available to males to prove themselves is to work harder and longer than anyone else. So men come to work earlier, work harder, and stay later than their peers. Some men use work as an escape from their spouses' desire for intimacy. Since these males are uncomfortable with emotional closeness, it becomes convenient to avoid it by working long hours. Sooner or later, however, they will pay a price for neglecting their bodies, not getting enough exercise, not eating properly, and not getting enough rest.

Oᴜᴛ ᴏғ Tᴏᴜᴄʜ

People are out of touch with their bodies because they are uneasy about sexuality. The guilt visited upon us by a repressive, misguided theology keeps us segmented and divided. There is conflict between spirit, mind and body. We are at war with ourselves. This robs us of a deep and satisfying spirituality because it is contrary to the way we were created. Only through an acceptance of our wholeness as creatures of God can we come to spiritual fulfillment. Complete acceptance of our bodies is possible only when we view our physical self as holy, as ordained by Jesus.

Gᴇᴛ Iɴ Tᴏᴜᴄʜ

In order for you to celebrate your sexuality, you will need to get in touch with your body. You will recall in the chapter on intimacy you were invited to look at your body. You may benefit from performing the practices outlined there at this time. When you do them a second time, you should become a little more comfortable with yourself. To really know your body you will need to become aware of the sensations it can experience. It is valuable to heighten our awareness of our senses, because this increases the pleasure we can experience.

Hᴇᴀʀɪɴɢ

Give attention to your hearing, think about what sounds are your favorite. Music is a natural thing to consider at this point. If you listen mainly to hard rock, break out of your rut! Try listening to some mood music and, if you can make the leap, there is a lot of beautiful classical music available. Nature's sounds are also very enjoyable. The chirping of birds and the songs they give us are a gift from God. Don't miss them! The sounds of other animals such as wolves, coyotes, and sheep can also be relaxing and life enhancing.

SMELL

Be aware of the smells you enjoy. One obvious area is perfumes and colognes. Women, select a perfume that heightens your sexual desirability. Choose what you like, but get feedback from others as to what goes well with your body chemistry. Learn to use the correct amount of perfume. Some women put on so much that when you get near them, it seems as if their scent could knock you over. What you wear should be subtle, intriguing. If it is too obvious and can be smelled 100 yards away, it is not nearly as sexually interesting to a man.

Men, choose your cologne with care. Find one with a good match for your body chemistry. Use the right amount. If you put on an excessive amount, you are the male version of the over-perfumed woman whose scent can stop traffic from all four directions. Experiment until you know how much is enough. Men also need to be aware of the hair tonic they use. Some of these hair dressings have very distinctive smells. I have been around men who have an overpowering smell emanating from their heads. In the presence of someone like this, you can scarcely get your breath. Most women will find this unpleasant, to say the least. Again, moderation is the key; don't use too much.

While we are on the subject of smells, I want to say a word about personal cleanliness. If you are going to be at optimum desirability in the eyes of your lover, it is important to be clean. Take a bath or a shower before you get romantic. Good hygiene also includes the inside of your mouth. Brush and floss your teeth. Not only will this improve your love life, it will also give you better dental health.

TASTE

Another very important sense is taste. Kisses have a taste to them; it is your lover's way of tasting you. If you brush and floss your teeth, your mouth will taste much better. I'm sure you are all familiar with the advertisements for the mouth-wash to banish "morning breath." Interestingly, if you brush and floss your teeth at night, you don't have "morning breath." You can add to the pleasure of your lovemaking by introducing other tastes into the process. Because of its almost universal appeal, chocolate is a good bet. You can place chocolate sauce on your lover's back and lick it off. This is a very sensual experience and tastes good, too! You can then progress to putting it on each others nipples and remov-ing it with your tongue. From there, the chocolate vagina and penis are a logical step. Enjoy!

Touch

Now we come to the most important sense in your sexual life: touch. Through touch you had the first sensual experience of your existence. It is how you first knew the world. Nursing at your mother's breast provided you with a flood of sensations. First, you touch her breast with your mouth and felt the vel-vet softness as part of your erotic experience. Then your taste buds were rewarded by the warm milk you drank from her body. She talked gently to you, maybe even sang a song to you, so your sense of hearing brought you peace and pleas-ure. Your mother also held you and this was comforting for both of you. This gives you some idea of the importance of touch in communication between and among human beings.

I have met people who have various ways of responding to touch, as I am sure you have. On the one end of the spectrum are those who touch freely. Once you have established rap-port with them, and this sometimes happens within a matter of seconds, they feel free to touch you, on the arm or the shoulder or some other neutral place. Touchers are pleasant to be around, at least for me, because it is easy to feel con-nected to them. They are generally open and interesting peo-ple with a lot of life in them. At the other end of the continuum are people who do not like to be touched. This type of person often refers to a toucher as a "touchy-feely person." This phrase generally reveals discomfort with touch, and therefore intimacy, on the part of the one who utters it. If you are one of these people, I urge you to enter into therapy and overcome your fear of touch. You are missing so much in life by avoiding tactile contact with your fellow human beings. You also will never reach the deepest intimacy with another if you cannot touch and be touched comfortably.

MASSAGE

One of the best ways to nurture your relationship is through massage. The communication you will have with each other via this medium cannot be achieved in any other way. By allowing your love to manifest itself through your hands, you bring together body, mind, and spirit. Your whole being is present in giving to your partner. When you are receiving a massage, love flows into you and fills you up. This is why an experience with your lover will always be better than one with a masseur/masseuse who is a stranger to you.

You may say you don't know anything about massage, so how are you going to give a good one? Go to the library and check out some books on the subject. When you are working with your partner, be creative, try new things. When you are receiving the gift of touch in this way, talk about what you like and don't like. Say it in a nice way, but communicate your wishes and desires to your lover. Don't rush the process, a massage may take around 30 minutes to be satisfying. If you are both going to be the beneficiaries of this sensual, nurturing, spiritual event, it could require an hour or more. Some couples make love either before or after, and this may take another hour. For the whole event, you may need two hours. This may seem like a long time, but consider the purpose of your activity. You are nurturing the most important part of your life, the relationship between you. Often we use two hours to go to a movie or sporting event and think nothing of the time invested, yet we are hesitant to devote the same length of time to our partner. You might want to examine your priorities if this is a problem for you.

PUTTING IT ALL TOGETHER

To really celebrate your sexuality, try combining all of the elements I have talked about. Decide on what music you want to play during your ultimate evening. Be aware of the way you smell and how your lover smells. Be clean and then put on some perfume and or cologne to enhance the experience. Brush your teeth, use mouthwash in addition to brushing if it helps increase your confidence. Decide what to wear. As a woman, you may wear a negligee or "teddy." As a man you may wear tight underwear or a robe. Give consideration to taste. I talked about using chocolate; if this doesn't fit for you, perhaps a certain beverage will improve the atmosphere. This can be alcoholic or non-alcoholic. If it is alcoholic, do not drink an excessive amount or it will impair your sexual performance. If you choose chocolate or some other flavor, be creative with it. Apply it to different areas and lick it off. Make sure there is mutual consent to all of your activities.

Candlelight will always enhance the romantic atmosphere. The flickering flame is a lot like our love as humans. Sometimes it is stronger and sometimes it is weaker. Touch one another in an uninhibited way. Massage your lover's body. Allow yourself to receive pleasure, surrender control, and let the experience engulf you. Do not hurry the event, let it unfold slowly. Talk to each other, let your lover know what you enjoy. Be present in spirit, mind, and body. Devote yourself to the other person, let go of any and all anger toward your partner. Your spirits will flow together if you let down the walls. Make love, enjoy the total connection between the two of you. Be aware of your spiritual, emotional, and physical union. Feast upon the deep communion you are part of, longed for by everyone, but denied to many. Let your heart overflow with thankfulness. Be grateful for your creation as a sexual being, know in the center of your being who you are. Become free of any guilt visited upon you by bad theology, whatever the source. Acknowledge God's divine wisdom in creating you in a way that enables you to come together in total union.

CLIMAX

Through your journey of lovemaking, you will come to the peak of orgasm. Be totally open to this sublime moment, with gratitude for the way you were created and for your lover. When your partner has her or his climax, enjoy it vicariously. Be glad for the other person, allow yourself to be close in spirit to the other. Be joyful in giving to your lover; sense the oneness in your relationship. After this, glory in your own orgasm. Let the sensation flow over you, join with your lover and with God in this great thrill of your existence.

SONG OF SONGS

As I am sure you have gathered by now, you have my full endorsement for a complete and satisfying sex life. Now I want you to accept the same support from the Word of God. In the Bible, from the Song of Songs, we can all learn about the enjoyment of sexuality. You and your lover may wish to read this book to each other. I will quote from Chapter 4; verses 1-6.

> *"How beautiful you are, my darling!*
> *Oh, how beautiful!*
> *Your eyes behind your veil are doves.*
> *Your hair is like a flock of goats descending from Mount Gilead.*
> *Your teeth are like a flock of sheep just shorn,*
> *Coming up from the washing.*
> *Each has its twin; not one of them is alone.*

Your lips are like a scarlet ribbon,
Your mouth is lovely
Your temples behind your veil are like the halves of a pomegran-
ate.
Your neck is like the tower of David, built with elegance, on it
hang
a thousand shields all of them shields of warriors.
your two breasts are like two fawns,
like twin fawns of a gazelle that browse among the lilies.
Until the day breaks and the shadows flee,
I will go to the mountain of myrrh and to the hill of incense."

Here is another quote from Chapter 7; verses 7-9.

"Your stature is like that of the palm and your breasts like clus-
ters of fruit.
I said, 'I will climb the palm tree, I will take hold of its fruit.'
May your breasts be like the clusters of the vine,
the fragrance of your breath like apples,
and your mouth like the best wine."

We see in this quotation a joyous appreciation of sexuality. The author is free to "take hold of its fruit." In other words to take hold of the woman's breasts. We are given the same freedom to enter into the enjoyment of the sensual experience of touching as lovers.

Christian teaching all too often has segmented us as humans and has contributed to people being cut off from their feelings and emotions, particularly men. It has divided the life of the spirit, mind, and body from one another. This has brought about a great amount of destructive behavior. One of these behaviors is rape. A man who sees the sexual act as a spiritual journey, nurturing both his lover and himself, could never rape a woman.

When more of us come to see lovemaking as the coming together of two people in a spiritual, emotional, and physical whole, we will have progressed as a society. More people will have had a deeply spiritual experience and this will stay with them until they die.

You were created as a sexual being. The Song of Songs provides a ringing approval of your existence as a sexual being. The Word of God itself gives you the freedom to be yourself. You may fully become involved in the great physical sensations of lovemaking. Be at peace with your body and recognize your wholeness as a person.

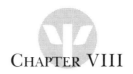

CHAPTER VIII

WORDS TO MAKE LOVE BY: LOVE POETRY

THE MOUNTAIN

Going up step by step, holding hands
intimately.

Looking into your beautiful eyes, sensing
peace and serenity there, silently singing
hallelujahs in your presence.

Reaching the top, holding you in the
warm sunlight of our lives with the shadows
far away.

Kissing your lips, tasting the flow of our
passion. Being aware only of this moment,
this spot of earth, and you.

Watching you undress in the full glory of
bright sunlight with total freedom, as nature and
God intended.

Reveling in the visual wonder your nakedness
presents to me. Praise to God comes out of my soul
for being here at this moment!

Undressing without awareness of my actions,
focused upon you and my good fortune in having
met you.

Lying with you on a blanket of clothes. Touching
and being touched in the grassland of the universe.

Sounds of passion in our embrace, excitement growing, penis growing. Mounting tension, mounting you, cries of ecstasy!

THE SHOWER

Soaping your breasts, touching them more than is
necessary to wash them. Watching the small
waterfalls carry away the bubbles excites me.
Your nipples, so pink and erect, speak to me of
oneness.

The foam on your derriere, the beauty of your
wonderful curving body, may hands sliding smoothly
over your spirit.

Your hands on my chest bringing to life my nipples,
softening my chest hairs with the touch of intimacy.

Touching your most private part, water and soap
flowing over the soft moist hair, like the love
flowing over this moment with a feast for my senses
and
spirit.

Your fingers upon my erection with the rush of
cleansing pleasure.

Our bodies in the embrace of freedom and giving.
A touching, a place of sacred communion of two
souls.

MOONLIGHT

Lying beside you in bed. The rhythm
of your breathing lifting the sheet with your
breasts.

Moonlight upon your face, playing with the
shadows, letting your loveliness burst forth.

Upon the breeze your unique perfume,
natural, sensuous, comes to me, whispering
the love song, filling my life with peace.

Moving toward you, touching your body,
coming to you with all of me, to merge with
all of you.

THE RAIN AND THE FIRE

Walking in light mist hands and hearts clasped.

Leisurely pace in tune with nature.

Suddenly sky opens, torrent of wetness upon us,
dashing to house, inside quickly, laughing,
heavy breathing, drenched clothes, slight chill.

Fire started, soggy garments removed,
toweling down, sensuous touching, desire rising,
blanket in front of fire, lights out, passion on.

Flickering light, bursting fireworks,
descending from the peak to the warm valley below.

Bathrobes on, hot cider with a shot,
warmth of fire and security of love.

All is serene.

A SENSE OF TOUCH

Soft skin played with the fingers, open and vulnerable.

Lotion spreading over your body, a pool of sensuality created in the shadows of love.

Firmness in the touch descending into tissue. Audible sounds of joy from your throat welling up into a song of love. The excitement of intimacy in our bond, wanting to nurture this above all else.

Coming to you with all my passion, unveiling the mystery of union between two children of God.

PLAYFULNESS

Sitting beside you, our bodies touching, hearing
your thoughts, rolling them over in my mind.

Giving them a new twist or slant, hearing the lilting
notes of your laughter, borne upon the breeze of our
shared happiness.

Pure joy between us, our hearts open to take it in.

being fully alive, seeing the smile on the divine
face as God shares in the revelry.

Free to travel life's road in the sunlight of love.

All made possible by seeing the humor in life.

Love Streams

In the woods of
spiritual renewal
sitting on the banks
of the river of Life
Kissing, nibbling first,
then with passion.

Removing the barriers
between us, material
and psychological.

Plunging into the cold water
letting exhilaration in.
Surfacing together, you
with bright pink nipples
alive with sensuality.
Excitement rushes into me
and I embrace your loveliness.

Leaving the water,
drying our bodies.
Settling onto a blanket
Coming together with our
deepest needs exposed.
Becoming one with each
other and with all of
Creation.

DOVES

Two white doves
gliding across the pond
of moonlight
Through the shadows
bobbing slightly
Speaking of sensuality
and ecstasy

Suspended above me,
barely touching my chest
The fruit of love
Ready for harvest
Gently caressed
by hands and lips

Gathering the bounty
into my life
with pure enjoyment
Becoming aware of the
Divine Plan for
the union of humans
in the most natural
of actions.

ONE WITH YOU

Let me warm my
soul in the fiery passion
of your love.

Touching your being
at the inmost place.
Holding you in the center
of my life as I am
held in the center of yours.
Leaving behind the cares
of the world for these moments.
Immersed in the sea
of union, safe within and
without.

SIMPLY LOVE

Fading light

Dark of night

Candles glow

Passions grow

Bodies meet

All's complete

Your comments on this work are welcome.
Please write or e-mail:

Beaver's Pond Press
5125 Danen's Drive
Edina, Minnesota 55439-1465

comments@beaverspondpress.com